Your Better Half (B2),
The art of the ART

Table of Contents

1

Format of Book

2/7/6/18
The Format/ Ground Rules for this book and
suggested method of reading with the
attached videography and how the reference
most effectively use these are as follows:

Video references have extensively appeared
in my books since my first book, "It's the
Liver Stupid," now in its 5th edition. The
video format has somewhat changed and
expanded over this some fifteen year or so,
especially since a great deal more of the
current applicable science is now available
on You Tube.

Today, virtually any topic whether
mainstream or radically controversial is now
offered on You Tube. The author has also
included much of his work, especially
experimentation there, but also it is used to
defend the totally new, ground-breaking
historic discoveries not commonly known as
well as scientific discoveries and current
breakthroughs that are just emerging.
Furthermore, they cover a few significant,
ground breaking, and yet unpublished,
discoveries that others have recently proven,
but are not peer reviewed.

Finally, if little of the rest of remaining
video is significant in itself, but one key
3

point serves to establish something that the author sees as a key reference, the beginning point of that reference is noted in italic parenthesis as *(9).* So *(9)* indicates that the key point is 9 minutes into the video. Further, if there are several other key point in an otherwise less significant video, those will be noted following the first to save you time. In every case, the author has viewed the entire presentation at least once. Rarely, a video will be used multiple times for multiple references, where they fit, to establish other key points.

Keep in mind that books will always outlast You Tube videos and you will have to reestablish any links lost yourself unless a newer edition is published. The attempt here is to provide enough information to do that, but at times, this is impossible.

Today, my first edition of "It's the Liver Stupid," today has very few live links left and many have been lost or have changed within just a few years. This book, "Your Better Half: or what I term "B/2" uses this format more often than any previously. To use it effectively, you must be at least use a handheld computer or cell, but seldom do you need a very large screen to get the point of these references and mostly the audio is important.

4

The Bibliography is kept very short, but does given some references to other work.

Book Outline and Points

B/2 documents a proven, powerful Age Reducing Therapy (coined ART herein) that virtually no one realizes is even an option today: That is say, Aging versus this ART is a true option for every person... Something that people have discussed for years as a fairy tale myth, but something that Newtonian science has begun to even recognize as a possibility with Teleomeres (which are very likely effects as reported and addressed later here). The proven facts reviewed herein (really a series of sometimes seemingly unrelated facts), that I pull together to establish my thesis is that we are infinite beings with very long possible lifetimes as advanced in topics, videos, and related commentary.

This is now documented history and proven science complemented by the work that my friend Dr. Price and I have done over the past fifteen years that I put into videos to allow you to experience it as reality. While no single element/ part of it proves it on its own, as a whole, it becomes a very compelling and I submit Written in Stone (fired clay tablets qualify), but the final proof, actually living it, will take thousands
5

of years to fully prove out. Maybe in two hundred years, some will start paying attention though as many begin living out the "Better Halves of Their Lives," and B/2 is a reality.

To begin this proof, I give you this short video on cancer with an interview by Raymond Francis, PhD Biochemical Engineer, Arthur, and Lecturer: https://www.youtube.com/watch?v=PcY1OandSf8

Here he lectures that cancer is not a disease, but is a reaction to toxins and diet, his two key issues. This I have always posited in my own books, but in very different terms and with, I submit, very different, but still valid and objective, arguments. Further, there is no conflict between what he teaches and B/2, the ART.

While I delve more deeply into this topic in my previous books, no one "gets" cancer who follows my suggestions and I give you cases where people have had "spontaneous remissions" as Alfred does follow my teaching. So, yes, Francis and I agree that cancer is not a disease and that it is a reaction to toxins and poor nutrition resulting in basic changes in cells. but I define disease differently than Francis.

Furthermore, my definition of human disease and in all of my books is that they are parasitic infections (I further define viruses and bacteria as micro-parasites). By my Merriam Webster dictionary, a disease is more narrow than either of us state, saying that its is, "Anything that impairs a vital function." Today, either definition is far too narrow when compared to current drug company usage. There, anything that can help sales is a disease and it has become an acronym in itself.

So with my definition of cancer: All parasites are biology and the are designed to thrive just as you are by nature. They commonly attack the weak where they can easily take up residence and multiply. Cancer with its necessary toxins and the compromised diet that generally precedes it weakens you, creating an ideal environment for parasites. I speculate that that parasites actually are what kill people with terminal cancer, but few ever live long enough today to allow that proof, since all cancer treatments will do the trick first.

Commonly, and we have good reason to believe this, given Royal Rife's work in the 1930's: With cancer, if you get rid of the parasites, the actual cancer condition will often revert to normal cell growth and the person will survive. This is pretty valid

7

proof that cancer does not actually kill anyone. There are obviously some rare exceptions where life functions cannot continue because, for instance, an organ is totally destroyed, but today, we just never reach this point. Keep in mind that a parasite that kills you destroys itself and nature is generally better than that at its game. The idea is to keep you alive as a host.

With the above in mind, let's begin with my premise here on the art of ART, our primary topic, as I teach you longevity and as I have reconstructed it from history, current, and cutting edge science:

The Scheme of B/2

B/2 does what we architects commonly do with projects. We create the basic design, known as "The Scheme," or Parti. Then, as project architect and designer, I assemble a team of experts. For buildings, they would consist of experts ranging from Structural Engineers to Land Surveyors.   In this case, I select a group of specialists like Raymond Francis, Biochemist, whose videos appear above and later herein. As with the Land Surveyors and Engineers, none of these as specialists would likely ever design a total ART solution individually as I do here, but each is very talented as a professional just as

8

Bruce Lipton, Raymond Francis and the
others are here.

With any project, I solidify the scheme into
a useful solution. That is, I develop the
scheme of parts into a working solution in
very much the same way that I designed B/2
and ART. This is exactly how all good
buildings are created and this is what B/2
does in its own unique way. No one speaker
or video contributor knows enough of the
history and science to formulate a B/2
solution himself or herself. Furthermore,
certainly, I do not know the individual
sciences or history well enough to tell a
complete story either and that would be
virtually impossible for one person to do.
However, I do know each part enough to
recognize its merits to formulate what I
consider a working solution or ART. In the
past, people referenced the books with a
bibliography and quoted the work of
readers. Compared to hearing them actually
tell their point of view, this is pretty weak in
my opinion. Also, how many people actually
read them and reference the work spelled
out?

So in B/2 the ART has a solid, proven basis
and nothing is fabricated from thin air, but
you as the reader must grasp all of the pieces
for it to work. Then you create an
"epigenetic working subconscious solution."
9

Without a thorough understanding of the parts, you cannot grasp this solution, so this will take a good deal of time and effort on your part, because you must know it well enough for your subconscious to accept and believe in. Videos help with this also. Teaching the subconscious as Bruce Lipton lectures is tricky, but once you grasp a topic well enough in this way, you are a part of the solution and it all comes together as an ART and works. Videos are more powerful than books, but the most powerful teaching technique is to live the experience, which is why you are here in this life, I suggest. Get these techniques down, live them, and tell others why you are young.

The above is to say that B/2 the ART does not start with a blank canvas, it starts with proven facts and it seeks to establish them so that you, a candidate for wellness, can live a long life and benefit. Other than the leap that established Newtonian science, a broad lie as Raymond Francis convincingly argues, you must take the final step to implement what is offered.

ART Aging Factors

Here in B/2, I point out in video documentaries that we have the true physical factors in hand that cause aging for the first
10

time in modern history where they are cohesively addressed. This is especially clear when the historically documented and scientifically observed facts are assembled that tell us that others in the distant part literally beat this aging that is now considered normal. With this, you see it all in B/2 and the results are in your face. I walk you through these in detail and you, of course, can disregard them (and die, as many will) or endorse them. Practice them, and live an extra half life (B/2) or possibly add thousands of years as others in the ancient past have done per proven records, with no exaggeration.

The above diversified factors not only keep you from aging, per my premise, they actually allow the de-ageing ART to occur both mentally and physically over time. Moreover, we are discussing a disease and pain free existence where you can make worthwhile contributions for a very long period... even longer than current written history. These contributions can overshadow anything you ever did previously in this first conventionally accepted part of life (you could term as B/1), as you move into "Your Better Half," (B/2) and much more.

Benefits of Longevity

11

I am not suggesting that our presently accepted short lifetimes are so bad, but obviously being sick and dying often is painful. However, when you have literally hundreds of years to pull off your life dreams, then those dreams actually have time to materialize into physical facts. Life's dreams do indeed take time to materialize. With long lives, you leave nothing for others to advance further or to lose through death. That is, in the past (and now), we simply did not live long enough lives to materialize most of our life dreams. Finally, very long life spans literally guarantee a great deal of spirituality and wisdom, if you are paying attention, and B/2 can help you learn to do that also.

My previous books have outlined how this de-aging can and has occurred, mainly through wellness, by directing you to the healthy tools needed to make them happen. With this B/2 writing, I assemble the toolbox giving you the place to further categorize your ART tools, but it adds a few powerful new ones in the process Even though aging is commonly regarded as a genetic predisposition by current science, this lie is dissolved with these ART facts.

Just from what you know at this point already, consider the absolute fact that aging is not a linear progression as Raymond

Francis says. Disease is an aging carrier just
as wellness is an ART factor in itself.
Francis is correct in saying that a cold ages
you and that all disease carries aging factors.
When you see a person with a cold generally
they look older. I suggest that this not an
illusion. They are, in fact, at least for the
time being aging... as my grandmother
would have said, "They are falling off.".
Finally, wellness is like carrying a bag of
wellness **beans** and each disease, in effect,
robs a small amount of beans for your bag.

Health Reversals in ART

Herein, I give you the observations and
proofs that health reversals are common and
have always occurred even within our
normally very short lifetimes today. Some of
these, you already commonly observe in
others, with such comments as, "You look
very good today." So, in fact, you intuitively
know much of this to be true by your own
daily observations, even though you may
disregard them long term. Yet this is almost
never taught or considered and is virtually
always disregarded by science today with
rare exceptions. Intuition is quantum science
at work. We all use it and even rely on it in
our daily lives. It relies on keen observation
and listening to our inner voice in response.

13

These above health reversals are in fact ART on a micro-scale. So the point here is that this ART can and does occur on a macro-scale. Now add to all of this, with Quantum Healing, aging at the microcellular level is quite reversible and telomeres can be lengthened as a part of this ART. Visually, ART is not so easy and the results take a fair amount of time to materialize. However, with the help of this extra mitochondrial energy production, the supplements, especially DMSO/MSM and those that I have pointed out in my previous books, give your exterior parts the tools to make you look younger and function more youthfully.

Aging is Good

Obviously, we want to continue to age chronologically of course. This allows us live and gain wisdom as I outline, but at the same time the idea is to de-age cellularly and biologically so as to even manifest those results as a youthful appearance, energy, voice, sight, etc as I address herein by topic. Antiaging is easier to accomplish, but ART absolutely makes it occur, and it must to some degree, as you recover from long term conditions which you may have even originated at birth as your cellular age is reduced.

Youth and Love

Now consider what Dr. Bruce Lipton
observes in his lecture here:

https://video.search.yahoo.com/yhs/search
?fr=yhs-pty-pty_email&hsimp=yhs-
pty_email&hspart=pty&p=You+tube+Br
uce+Lipton+Lovers#id=10&vid=2022ef4c
f5bc63d64c276845ad12ef67&action=view

People in love are virtually always young
and vibrant looking and acting, not just
because of what Bruce says, but because
their hormones and vibrations are peaked. In
fact, people in love seldom become ill. Love
is a building state that helps fill up your
bean bag just as being around young
children does. Kids literally teach the fact
that youth is a state of mind just as old age is
the opposite. For this reason, as you grow
older, the last thing that you want to do is
live in a retirement home with the dying to
play bingo and bridge. Here, your bean bag
is essentially emptied completely, you are
no longer making a contribution to society,
and you have cashed in all of your chips.
Your game is over and you are waiting to
die, so death is a wish fulfilled.

Finally, as all of my books teach you to
avoid this useless state, but you must learn
15

the various forms of contemplation/
meditation. Furthermore, ten minutes a day
as Raymond Francis suggests is just not
normally enough to get rid of and neutralize
the mental build-up and stress common in
today's rat race. There may have been a time
when ten minutes was enough, but today,
no. In fact, everything that you do should
carry some of the love that you gather in
contemplation and going into it and out of it
must become a general habit throughout
your daily routine. It is a form of
daydreaming really and is quite natural.
Some days, I need hours to get rid of the
garbage and others only require ten minutes
those are infrequent.

The Hype
Commercial Antiaging Creams

Next, in the mainstream media, some so
called, miracle creams, etc, claim de-aging
complete with before and after proof. But, I
contend that there is no such cream on the
market today and this ART is a coordinated
event that must begin deep inside the cells at
the microcellular level inside and work its
way out as I describe herein. Topical skin
applications which should amount to
transdermal supplements, do have a place
here, but this ART starts at the microcellular
level and not at the outer skin surfaces. It all
shows up externally as hearing and sight

loss, skin wrinkles, and even slow nail and hair growth among others. If you appear to look younger on using dermal creams and applications, invariably, just like dying your hair, they will reverse. With most commercial creams, given their unregulated chemicals, there is a long term price beyo nd their commonly high cost to pay, and you will pay, since they are generally ill conceived and trivial. Finally, keep in mind that photo shopping youth does not make it real and being a movie star or rock singer does not help anyone learn to stay young, so why give them your attention?

Beneficial Aging Factors

With B/2, actual mental aging as outlined and is a part of the ART, as discussed herein, aging is a true "benefit" scientifically in itself. However, herein also, we see that other physical factors are associated with mental increases that parallel the physical factors such as improvements in blood plasma quality as well as full use of your brain which is key to all of this, things seldom if ever discussed, but proven by observation and reported here in B/2 later. So as an eighty year old youth, you now be prepared to enter the most productive period of your life, but the sooner you begin this preparation, the easier it is to make the

17

transition to these more robust years ahead
of you once you control the negatives.

To summarize this introduction: B/2
provides you the physical pathways to youth
starting at the mitochondrial level where the
hard work is all done as pointed out in my
earlier books, but expanded on herein as an
ART. Here, we open the door of the
quantum biology of life that is always
striving to keep you alive as most of the
more informed scientist now grasp. At the
same time, I teach that you really can de-age
your outer conditions also to augment the
quantum by working from the outside as the
skin, hair, eye, voice, tactile, smell, taste and
hearing (factors that commonly begin the
fail) begin to de-age to match these internal
raised functions, thus consolidating the
ART.

You are indeed a whole human organism.
When these outer benefits are expanded and
increase your health. They serve to convince
you subconsciously that this ART is a
winner. Keep in mind that the subconscious
is a huge part of the ART and without totally
convincing the subconscious mind, nothing
special can really occur.

Your Makeover

18

From an architectural viewpoint: The net
result of this ART is a total biological
makeover never before encountered in
modern times. These makeovers were
seldom required (maybe every 200 years) in
ancient times, but these were completely
normal and anticipated by ancient people.
To switch analogies (I am a trained
mechanic also): They occurred in much the
same way as you would have your car
serviced today or repaired after an external
collision, but never with surgery. The
makeover in ancient eras included hot baths,
monatomic gold, and other interventions just
as I allude to under my chapter on Hot Tubs.

As the architect, switching hats again, this
makeover is analogous to taking an old
house that has begun to fail and rebuilding it
from the frame up, and I use this illustration
often herein. In a makeover, you save the
pieces that are still functional, add new
parts as required and basically end up with
a new house in most respects. However, in
either a house makeover or a car restoration,
you save the valuable pieces and generally
keep the parts that give the house, car or
your human body character while adding to
it, making it more functional.

Even better than a makeover, just as in
ancient times, I give you the tools herein to
allow you to continually maintain your
19

house in new condition and always
functional once it is restored to peak
operation with the ART. In terms of your
biology, this allows you to recondition
systems before they fail on an ongoing basis,
making it essentially indestructible until you
step into a disastrous condition. No matter
what, life must end... you must eventually
die and there is no escaping it. At some
point, you will and must find a way to die,
but the point of the ART is to make it
happen on your terms if possible.

Who Benefits From B/2

But there is more. With the above,
hopefully, as a conscious Soul, you will gain
wisdom and love using the biological tools
that I give you and become more spiritually
advanced. These are the things that most of
us generally missed in our first half of life
(B/1) here at least to a great degree. When
we carry these qualities with us, our lives
are full of textures and nuances that the
youth starting out today are just not ready to
endorse or entertain and thus, where they
commonly fail. Chronologically, the youth
today simply do not have, and generally
never have had in the past, the gears or the
horsepower yet to go where I hope to open
the door with ART for you, this threshold
for you to cross. When you have sixty to
eighty-five years of hard knocks behind you,
20

you have the foundation, the ART to work for this total makeover. The biggest problem here is for you to surrender your past habits, unlock your full mind as you can as B/2, the ART, teaches, and get onboard. Then, the rest will be easy. Still if you are just forty of fifty years old, you have a good start on this journey to wisdom as you make this transition to a new youth, if you elect to do so, so this is a book for you also.

If you are just twenty or thirty years old, can you gain from this book? Of course, learn the ART first, but no one can tell you what is coming next as you grapple with the hard questions of life that await you (and generally only using half of your brain as B/2 tells you). You, as a relative youth will change a great deal mentally as we all do, as documented and I point out here, when they manifest as they must. Still, for you, this B/2 is a big heads-up that you can use to help save you plenty of headaches as you anticipate the coming enlightenment as these new facts roll out and they will. From here, my suggestion for you is to hang out with someone who has pulled this off this ART and emulate them. Wisdom and spirituality do rub off and their effects can be somewhat superimposed on you if you are open to them. That is, spirituality is caught and not taught as others have expressed. But you must be here and
21

prepared to catch it: Spirituality does not fly
out of the woodwork of old houses; And you
must be well enough in the process to
receive it. Indeed, there is a point of no
return. A very sick person seldom can focus
on anything but their disease and pain and
seldom does a deathly ill person ever make
much spiritual progress.

Forget Breakthroughs

Our present social focus on highly
technological breakthroughs is not going to
get you there either. I introduce you here in
B/2 to a few of the lies that you are told, but
they manifest throughout society today as
they pin their hopes on useless high
technology and drugs. You must take
personal responsibility for all that happens
to you for B/2 to be effective. The
ignorance dispersed by "modern" society is
not about to lessen anytime soon. This, even
though we are going through a
transformation that will eventually expose
our present social ills and technical
ignorance for what they really are. Melting
them away will take decades as the power
hungry loosen their grip on society and we
begin to see things more clearly. Along with
these also, the many illusions that surround
them such as fiat money must lose their grip
in this process.

Who We Are

So why did we miss this stuff before? First, our society has endorsed this very short lifetime, that relative to our genetic code, has been proven to be far shorter than the ancients and ends at seventy or eighty as normal. It also endorses quick turn arounds, fast cures, and fast money with these short lifespans. Still, after all, these aborted lifetimes have been considered normal and accepted now for several thousand years. Also, for current science to endorse it, there is no proof in the fossil record of long lifetimes (so science will not buy this easily), but that would be nearly impossible to expect as we learn herein for humans.

The assurance then, is that, as a population, we remain basically ignorant as we are killed off just as we begin to gain a degree of insight into the real scheme of things and to fathom just how life really works. In fact, today's seventy or eighty obviously equals that of an Annunachi teenager given that they live several thousand years. Now we know that they in fact did and this is documented and proven on clay tablets in ancient Sumarian/Mesopotamian's history... essentially, written in stone and still there today. Furthermore, our entire population today is at least half-bred Annunachi/ Mesopotamian in their genetic code. If you

23

are not versed on who the Annunachi are, watch the video below. It is only based on historic clay tablet information, but it is a start and very good proof. This secret is revealed as stone-cold fact herein. Nothing else this old is so certain in this world today and so well preserved.

Dowsing

This technique, commonly known as a pseudoscience among the Newtonians, has become very popular with Quantum (defined below) Scientists of today and it is becoming more accepted as we enter this new era even if it is subjective. Watch Dr. Bruce Lipton and Dr. Dan Nelson and others on You Tube who mainly use muscle testing as I discuss on this video:
https://video.search.yahoo.com/yhs/search ?fr=yhs-pty-pty_email&hsimp=yhs-pty_email&hspart=pty&p=You+Tube+James+Robert+Clark+Quantum#id=16&vid=7743a76623b5c6c7001a81003889adae&action=view

So how accurate is this dowsing? Test it yourself, but I have seen total 100% accuracy on the two occasions where I have carefully tested it on as plus/ minus with existing hidden conditions. If you do not come out so well, keep testing and learning

to apply it on the many seemingly
outrageous concepts, science, and history
introduced herein. Know how good you are
at any given time and keep testing your skill
as you improve. You actually have 99%
ability right now, but total accuracy comes
with experience and confidence. The
problems occur when you doubt your
ability. People have been using this to find
water in wells for hundreds of years as
scientist laughed at them. This is a part of
Qaantum Science and it is based on your
unconscious mind, which is far better than
your studied information and, as discussed
below, quantum must eventually dominate
our science.

Use this to test who you should be seeing for
a naturopath or doctor, or even what
supplements are good for your particular
body and who you should trust as a friend.
The applications are wide spread and
endless, and the time required to test
anything is fast. Also, you can retest
quickly to be certain. What was a good idea
yesterday can be a bad one for you today as
the situation surrounding it evolves and
changes. When you are really good at this,
you just know and actually testing it is not
required, but then it still is a useful
agreement. When you have this tool down
solidly, you will have mastered self-

awareness. Still, its always nice to have visual proof as confirmation.

Wellness In General

Let's continue with
https://www.youtube.com/watch?v=XExB
45GRrfc

This is a 2nd, longer, video by Raymond Francis, PhD, biochemist, and author on wellness, as he introduces the general basis of my thesis here and in my earlier books. His assumptions and points generally agree with what I point out here and began with in the pursuit of wellness. So I begin here with his presentation as a starting point and play off with comments on it:

Herein, Francis has hit on most every key beginning point that I make in all of my books and he is correct in pointing out that all disease is effectively based on toxins or cellular failure due to a lack of proper nourishment. But before getting into the meat of his talk, note that he does not consider parasitic diseases as I hear him. These are generally defined by the parasites that cause them like Lyme and Malaria, even though your immune system must be somewhat deficient for them to occur. I consider bacteria and viruses (all living

26

organisms) to be parasites also. An
extremely healthy body will not only ward
off parasites, it will not be affected by even
stings, mosquito, and even poisonous snake
bites (to my amazement). Basically, if you
are properly nourished and are free of many
toxins, nothing makes you ill, period. But
beyond that, you do not age and, in fact,
your cellular age decreases as a quantum
being. At the moment, I am nearly 76 and
my cellular age is 12 today, but it ranges to
17 commonly for various reasons, mostly
for me, it is too much or too little sleep that
changes it. Cellular age varies often with
toxin exposure, attitude, foods that you eat,
sleep, and exercise and for me, it varies 30%
from one day to another, so maybe next
week mine could be 17 again, but I get
plenty done when I sleep and this is the
price I pay occasionally.

Now, lets discuss Francis's more detailed
points:

Francis speaks of genetic signals, which is
epigenetics defined. Your attitude has a
huge age implication on wellness and when
you are upset, nervous, angry, or afraid,
your cellular age increases and the degree of
increase is often beyond anything
imaginable. A really bad car accident, for
example, might age you twenty years. If you
are already 80 and compromised, an
27

accident that a cellularly younger person might be just injured in easily could kill you.

With what I give you in this book when combined with "Its the Liver Stupid," will reduce the cost of disease to zero obviously, since I never am sick. This is true for everyone who follows what I outline. No one becomes diseased when they are using the ART that I introduce herein after a few years. So my smaller goal here is to cut the disease to zero while setting you up for a much longer lifetime than anyone today lives using this ART. With this, you must venture beyond what Francis considers, however, as there will be huge social and governmental problems attached to this as I point out here.

In order to do what I suggest, you must be pro-actively prepared not just actively. More comments on Francis' talk:

(9.6) Never focus on calcium in your supplements (I have written extensively on this in earlier books).

(10.4) He is very accurate on people craving food and weight gain as a result. Food craving is very common with pregnant women as we know. They are giving up valuable nutrients to a controlling fetus and thus have cravings for this same reason.

28

Since few get all of the essential nutrients needed for both themselves and the fetus, they come up short in some areas and typically they generally gain too much weight during pregnancy because of these deficiencies. Thus, both weight gain during pregnancy and weight gain in general are from a common cause, diet deficiencies.

(11.4) Notice that we do not need drugs to balance our systems. This is key.

(13.3) Francis suggests that all calories are the same... but not so. Toxins, by his definition, cause fat controls to be jammed. His is an interesting angle, but everyone in the alternative field generally knows that these "toxins" cause weight gain. As I walk through any supermarket, nothing there generally dowses as food in my experience, with very few exceptions. Dan Nelson points this out in his talk also. I disagree that animal protein, in itself, makes you gain weight. He does explain why some animal protein causes weight gain, but it is not the protein itself if you are listening.

All forms of arthritis go away when you follow my protocols and this is always the case. Using Francis' own analogy: Telling me that arthritis is not a disease does not cure it. Proper diet helps, but there is more to it. HL MSM and DMSO will cure all joint

29

problems. His suggestion are most likely very helpful, but there is more.

The basic unit of life is the cell, but, delving deeper, the key to wellness lies at the microcellular level, the mitochondria. The mitochondria are the center of your energy production and they are affected by HL MSM and DMSO in ways that no one even discusses or currently is aware today.

Saunas are excellent toxin removers to some degree, but herein I tell you about saltwater/ DMSO hot tubs which I believe must beat any sauna by miles. Salt water in itself is a huge contributor to health even when just sprayed on your body after a shower. So my hot tub solution will restore your minerals while removing toxins to an even greater degree.

(43) I suggest that light is sound vibration as discussed later herein, and that the cells are quantum devices. They communicate at speeds exceeding those commonly associated with either light or sound on the quantum level. In fact, they actually reverse time occasionally which means that events observed can be reversed and your age is reversible. Reversing disease is about allowing your body to do what it already knows it can do. and it starts at the mitochondrial level. Everything that
30

happens or has occurred does so objectively once you see the whole picture. Spiritual experiences do not erase time, but to the observer, they certainly appear to. Quantum space and time are fluid only because these laws change with time. Thus, this ART will change aging and its limits, just as subconscious agreement with current lies will kill you at age 80 or thereabouts.

Dr. Francis gets the "Basically Nonsense" "Stupid" part of my story and the even more "Unscientific Nonsense". His main points are totally accurate just as his comment that the cellular age of 10 year olds is commonly 45 today. My age, as I reported above, is somewhat flexible and I beat the common 10 year old today by at least 400%. I introduced dowsing earlier. You can measure your age using it to correlate his numbers, but you can do it quickly and much more cheaply. Finally, "How did modern medicine get the idea that feeding a person poison can make them well."

Dr. Francis tells us that his 100 year old car is "maintained" and that is why it is in excellent condition. Herein, I tell you how to provide additives using the ART to maintain new car condition and even how to make your car body over. Just as most of the cars that he relates to have been rebuilt and restored, I tell you how resoration is possible

31

for you also. The process may not be so deterministic as with machines, but the end result is equally impressive.

So reviewing the above: The reason that I start with Francis is that his key points parallel B/2 and in most ways, even though he never really considers the ART... how we can actually de-age beyond avoiding toxins and eating good food. Yet he virtually points out every step that B/2 hits on before it gets into the meat of the ART.

Sun Gazing and Exposure

Sun Gazing is one method of softening the pineal gland among its many other benefits that are never studied and not well known: https://www.youtube.com/watch?v=g85i2LdHrKw
The cover of B/2 is about Sun Gazing and Spirituality. As an architect, I always recommend ways of bringing the sun into your life. My "Cakes and Ale" spoken of above are most important at high noon with UVA & UVB with its higher wavelengths (vibrations) as it causes you to make vitamin D so essential to wellness. Go slowly and decide for yourself, but astaxanthin is a huge help here when dealing with excess. Dr. Mercola has lectured on this extensively, so listen to his presentations relative to Vitamin

D, but also how sunlight works to benefit
your health with its biological properties and
its vibratory spectrum in general. Mercola
and his guests are the experts, but lets
expand on what they say below:

B-Endorphins have, by this, been proven to
increase your sleep, happiness, and health in
many areas and in many ways. One thing,
for certain, is that sunscreens and sun
glasses block the beneficial sunlight. I
supplement D3 at 5,000IU summer and
10,000 IU winter daily and get maximum
sun exposure whenever possible. With that,
I look toward the sun without protection
whenever I think of it. I say this in many
places, but neither of these experts know
that astaxanthin will keep you from ever
being sunburned, so, despite popular
conceptions, a LOT of sunlight is good for
you.

https://video.search.yahoo.com/yhs/search
?fr=yhs-pty-pty_email&hsimp=yhs-
pty_email&hspart=pty&p=you+tube+dr.
+mercola+sunlight#id=2&vid=caaf2d716
17d338a1f72b61ae61fdced&action=view

The video below is now a very old one
(2013) in terms of what has been discovered
in science recently as presented above, but it
has merit:

33

<u>https://www.youtube.com/watch?v=
zjf_URaDTRY</u>

If you missed any of the first reference above
video skip through and review it again and
watch the whole thing with Calvin Howard
Especially *(10)* and *(1:03),* Howard is wrong
about why no hurricanes, but that is a topic
of another book. Hurricanes begin within the
internal earth vibrations and my friend
Nathan Rogers shut those events down in
the year that he observed no hurricanes.
Nathan who helped develop the CP4U and
earlier the concept that led to his absolute
control of hurricane events, but your
government is not interested. He even
offered to give his technology to NASA, yet
we still have hurricanes today.

(1:10) The sun is a vibration and it is not
hot. It becomes hot when its microwave
vibrations hit the atmosphere. This argument
has been around for forty years and it may
be true, but the point is well taken.

UV is absolutely beneficial to your health
and sunglasses are a detriment as Dr.
Alexander Wunsuch, MD points out below:

34

Virtually all that Wunsuch reports here is known to alternative medicine. The reason that he makes B/2 is that he is a German Doctor and has determined these facts on his own, to his credit. Furthermore, he is passionate about what he has found and recognizes that what he has observed is in total conflict with what science currently teaches regarding sunlight and its affects on our bodies.

Finally, I find his illustrations impressive and revealing if you have not gotten this elsewhere previously. What he does not know is that astaxanthin absolutely protects us from sunburn and he still discusses sunscreens and lotions as reasonable, responsible ways to stop sunburns. My own findings has proven, without a doubt, that sunburn nearly is impossible after you have taken astaxanthin for just two months.

Given the beneficial sun affect, we need to get at least 1/2 hour of sun at high noon every day when possible and UV light is extremely beneficial to both eyes and skin. Finally, I use DMSO full strength on my eyelids and face daily along with astaxanthin cream and it supplements sunlight.

Solar Food

As my first book pointed out, the idea is to eat raw food as much as possible and as Dr. Aris Latham points out, cooking food is really uncooking it and raw foods are the most nutritious since they basically bottled up sunlight and cooking reduces the contained solar energy:.
https://www.youtube.com/watch?v=oTp WUmJw4O4

Unfortunately, the sound quality is very poor on this video and it drifts, but it one of the most important presentations on raw foods that you are likely to find anywhere as it accurately categorizes vegetables and tells you how they work with your body. Dr. Latham is the most comprehensive person that I have ever heard on this topic. To outline it is difficult if not impossible, but he appears to miss very little.

Let me be clear, Latham is a confirmed vegan and I hold that this is inefficient. Still, meat today in our stores is generally full of toxins. but so are our vegetables. So to discredit animals as a dense food source, is inefficient.

36

It Really is a Toxin Story

Fresh foods are the answer with no or few toxins. We can deal with a few toxins and our livers are biologically equipped to do that. Overwhelm your liver and the autoimmune system is overwhelmed. An overwhelmed liver is expressed as cancer just as a heart with insufficient blood supply is a expressed as a heart attack. Again, plants, especially store bought, are full of toxins. Eating a lot of anything poisons your body because there are so very few clean food choices today.

So lets consider first the toxins:

- Commercially grown vegetables
- Most tap water
- Commercial skin care products
- Beef, Pork, and Poultry
- Most all packaged foods

Now the clean energy sources:

- The Sun
- Our filtered Living Water
- Garden vegetables home grown

Sources with fewer toxins:

- Very small fish (as in sardines).
- Goat meat

37

- Coconuts
- Goat whey
- Moringa leaf
- Cacao
- Taurine

Research other ways to eat and drink with low toxic intake, but your choices are very limited. In fact, there is no vegan or meat solution in most grocery stores. Dr. Latham is good.

HRM's report

This man was tested by scientists and has not eaten for twelve years. He is thus free of toxins because his liver can easily deal with any that he breaths or absorbs. This would mean that his body is over 100% efficient, since he is living, moving, and talking. He is living proof that his body is a quantum machine that thrives on solar vibrations. You can assume that he is something very special, but so are you!

There are and always have been masters on earth who never eat/ate food, so HRM is far from unique. However, the spiritual masters are not here to prove anything and until you have evolved to a high spiritual level you will likely never know who they are.

HRM is claiming to use solar energy to run his body. If so, he is not really at the 100% level, but let's not split hairs, he is doing very well. He obviously knows a few things spiritually and, importantly, he has the attention of Newtonian Scientists in this 2012 video. I expand on what he is saying below.

Sun Gazing as reported below is available to all of us. HRM does project a good deal of wisdom here, but there is more, beyond what he is telling us. In fact, no one can tell you about spirituality. He knows it, but the requirement is to pass on what you are given and a few will catch it.

Quantum Defined

To begin, lets define one of the basic terms used often here and in previous books. Obviously, as you would expect, the definition here is not likely to conform with those of mainstream science, but I submit that very few of them are dealing with it beyond the popular two slit experiment that is currently overwhelming scientists to day. They know happens every time and they must acknowledge it, but it literally destroys all that they previously were taught. Note that current scholars attempt to put quantum science is a box as a micro scale

39

event. But sorry folks it occurs at every scale. I have an experiment on plants running on it as I write this.

Virtually all scientists in this transition are totally amazed that their high tech two slit experiment can apparently "read your mind." With this, they are mired in several thousand years of mind sets and a Newtonian lie that refuses to go away even as their core beliefs are discredited on a daily basis. In actual application, you are made up of trillions of cells and each one thinks and reports to your conscious mind instantaneously as they work to keep your body working as a unit. Your body, then, is a brilliant quantum computer and it is self healing when you rely on its inherent abilities. The real topic here is that as a quantum device, you are unlimited, but we will come back to that.

Adding to the above: by my observations, anything that anything that is quantum, is either biological in origin or is working under a similar system rules and it is not at all scale sensitive.

Quantum V Binary

Lets begin by comparing for instance, today's binary computer systems to Quantum Computing:
40

Quantum Computing and other quantum systems, when they function, literally think and draw in information intuitively just as do our CP4U chips do on cars and cause plants to grow faster as I report on elsewhere in my books.

This quantum model is in no way like the binary systems that we selected for computing up till now. Instead of adding up zeros and ones, Quantum systems adjust and learn just as your body does. Furthermore, Binary systems shift code at very high speed and possess no inherent intelligence. They learn on microchips, which I was shocked to discover are truly decapitated and thus ignorant lab crystals. We came to learn this, to my absolute amazement, while working with them on cars Full grown 8" lab crystals actually can learn and adjust to changing conditions and they commonly do. Indeed, given the opportunity, they are true quantum devices, but once they are slivered off they have no such abilities. I wonder what brilliant scientist figured this out and was he subversive in doing it?
https://video.search.yahoo.com/yhs/search?fr=yhs-pty-pty_email&hsimp=yhs-pty_email&hspart=pty&p=You+Tube+James+Robert+Clark+Cp4U#id=2&vid=587fca6c189837e17ce3cead9b768a64&action=click

Binary systems must reduce all information to a series of ones and zeros. Obviously, such a systems is extremely wasteful and absolutely the opposite of your biological mind, which is actually totally efficient even as the quantum system is currently misunderstood by today's science.

Nevertheless, we have managed to make binary, linear computing useful despite its wasteful origins and pitfalls. Furthermore, these decapitated microchips over these past thirty years of so-called progress have done quite a lot of good work. You could easily equate this struggle in computing progress to our internal combustion engines in many ways as both started with inherently flawed technology and methods. Over time, our own quantum mind with its intuition and creativity worked with them and made them useful, which teaches just how good we are.

As I posited in my first book, "Its the Liver Stupid" "your mind is a quantum device." In current QC work, QC is incorrectly said to rely on what they term as cubits of information. However, the science is new and just getting started and I submit that they simply have their concepts wrong. Our mind intuits information globally in ways that science cannot possibly fathom, but that QC world must eventually begin to approximate. Today, QC is certainly in it
42

infancy and not nearly where it must be developed to equal that of the Annunaki systems of even 80,000 years ago. Still, we are beginning with QC from a proper starting point even if our understanding is currently flawed. These flawed systems must go by the wayside as we move forward in this new era.

Certainly, QC, in its final form will no longer require nearly absolute zero temperatures as obviously your mind, our CP4U, and advanced Annunaki systems do not. https://video.search.yahoo.com/yhs/search?fr=yhs-pty-pty_email&hsimp=yh However, we have indeed begun the Quantum Computing (QC) era, even if we are not close to where it must quickly develop.

This video glance below speaks to where it will progress on this pathway. It may be dead wrong, but it is referenced here to help you realize just how far off we have been up till now: https://www.youtube.com/watch?v=CMdHDHEuOUE Obviously, NASA, in this video is way off base as it commonly is. Anything described as biological, by today's science is really a huge problem, since our science is still generally locked into

43

Newtonian concepts that have never truly
applied to our the real world.

Quantum Biology

This, new to this era, is a huge topic, and
many books can and will be written on it.
Furthermore, it can be expanded to include
anything that has lived or is living today.

Now that current science is forced to
entertain truth, even though through very
dark glasses, the reality is that everything
that exists in biology is again quantum
science and this has always contradicted
what Newtonian Science just cannot fathom.
Furthermore, biology will remain a huge
mystery as long as it serves as the basis for
any part of our viewpoint given current
science hang-ups.

When you accept this basis, that you are a
Quantum Machine, then you realize that
current science has always been a huge lie
and can never rise above such lies with the
pharmaceutical industry, oil companies, etc
as its commercial starting points. Nicola
Tesla and his "Wheelhouse of Nature," was
another way of referencing the energy of
natural systems and biology that begin to
reveal the truth that we still manage to
circumvent and avoid for the most part

44

today, yet a few have learned to hear after one hundred wasteful years of so called progress. But Nicola Tesla was excommunicated from our current science/ religion even before he died and today most even consider along with that, Thomas Edison as the inventor of electricity. With what occurred with Tesla, all of science decided that it was the money that was important, not facts, and since then very few facts have been allowed to creep in as they were mostly shoved to the wayside for money.

If you watch what my friend Rich and I discovered initially with the CP4U and cars below:

https://www.youtube.com/watch?v=xm34 6TwkAhQ

It begins with the fact that all machines today are at best 30% efficient and few are that good. Science claims that your body is not any better than its ignorant machines and this is commonly reported and, yes, we in fact, commonly waste a good deal of what we eat, but in its defense, our food is garbage to the Annunachi. To start with food and digestion as a measure of your body's efficiency is a misrepresentation of what is biologically occurring and what can occur. At the cellular level, your mitochondria are essentially 100% efficient

45

when allowed to be and at times likely far exceed measurable unity.

Quantum Virtual Reality Computing (QVRC)

Adding Virtual reality to the up and coming QC process will have many benefits and one will be that it will point out this observation that you this Quantum Machine are unlimited in your potential and are not subject to lifespans.

QVRC is a gradual process, but one of the most powerful tools ever from a spiritual viewpoint. This technology will help us move all of this forward as we see the advent of true QVRC. From the more mundane viewpoint, this new Quantum Computing (QC) era, as reported below, will dispose of computer viruses and passwords, the bane of current computer generation. In the process, it will add many times the power currently available:
https://video.search.yahoo.com/yhs/search?fr=yhs-pty-pty_email&hsimp=yhs-pty_email&hspart=pty&p=youtube+quantum+computing#id=2&vid=c6c7c1e3735f86cdf4145ee75464308b&action=click

Keep in mind with the above, that these systems are flawed and technically limited

46

but very useful. As you may guess, they are
missing some key components and the
above report is totally ignorant as to where
we are headed with this technology. This
technology is straight from the Annunachi,
however, and QC has been in place for
many thousand of years with them as the
clay tablets of Sumaria report fairly clearly.

But QC is just about to occur here on earth
again. Once it does, this QVRC will allow
us, for the first time to emulate the profound
Annunachi systems and these breakthroughs
that they commonly used will not require
these nearly absolute zero temperatures
(check it out through dowsing as I teach).
The result will be true virtual reality systems
that will accommodate virtual biology and
morph systems that will make the robots of
Star Wars look like our current M1 army
tanks. With this, you will be able to virtually
visit friends world wide and do everything
except truly mate with your wife and
impregnate her. No, sperm and vaginas are
already operating at the quantum level and
there will never be a possibility for
improving them. Read my book, "Pretty
Fine Sex is Spiritual" for more on this topic.

QC and Diagnosis

Furthermore, the QC systems when fully
developed will be extremely compact (again,
47

check me out here and dowse it) and they will be very useful in the diagnosis of diseases, virtually eliminating the need for our harmful present radiology/ x-rays. Moreover, you will be able to wear a QC that is less cumbersome than a pair of sunglasses and will interface with us directly through your eyes and mind with no external device such as a mouse, voice or touch. Finally, its speed will be equal to your normal biological systems by definition, which in some ways is infinite and thus unlimited.

The main headache here is that everyone currently believes that QC requires near absolute zero temperatures and they are disregarding the fact that our minds are quantum machines. Once they learn to model the QC on actual biological systems, these lies will evaporate and we can move on to the really great solutions in store as did the Annunachi. Thus far, they are trying to reach into their past technology that relied on the binary code that is virtually unrelated. Doing this is analogous to repairing a jet engine using internal combustion engine technology.

Keep in mind that our earth people are simply behind. We do have the intelligence and we can and will pull this off, but QC is a technologically huge step and will teach us spiritual lessons beyond anything ever known as it points out the obvious facts that we currently chose to ignore as follows:

QVRC is Spiritual

Most importantly, all of this is occurring at the quantum/ spiritual level. The changes will be incremental as this QC technology improves and it really is not so highly technical. Currently, QVRC is at a rudimentary level here today primarily in gaming and porn applications. Once fully implemented, however, it will seem very normal and easy to grasp with no complex program instruction, unlike what we deal with presently. If you are aware and listening, you will catch these improvements as they reveal themselves, but the entire computing industry is being transformed.

In this transition, conversely, if you are sleeping and continue to endorse mainstream drugs and government backed technology, you are going to start becoming ill at age fifty and die with the general population somewhere around seventy or eighty. Also, chances are that your last ten years will literally be hell, as is currently the norm and you will be in pain even though you may not even remember what has occurred and this is also going to remain the norm also during this transition.

49

How QVRC Relates to Your life

The true and by far most important spiritual
key here is that QVRC will teach you
through simple, understandable reality
lessons that you observe "first-hand" that
life itself is a virtual reality system... that
you do not die ever and you are never killed
off in one lifetime, This key lesson here
then, is that nothing stops. You are a
continuation, simply with a new body and
you just start over. With each lifetime, the
biology may be new, but you carry within
you the lessons and memories of all past
lifetimes. These are never lost. You are
often, born into the same family group as
before. Seldom is anything totally new, but
the rules are flexible. One simple rule is that
you switch sexes to help maintain balance.
What is the lesson here? Treat the opposite
sex well, because you will become that,
next lifetime and your skin color could
change. The reality of our present computer
games and VR is just far too low to teach
any of this, but when we end up with
10,000,000 times the present computer
power, even these will become totally real
and help to drive this point home in ways
that you cannot imagine.

With computer games, you will be allowed
to fight wars and kill people. But do not
50

believe that just because society will allow
that that, there is no payment. The same
basic rules will apply as with dreams. When
you dream that you are killing a person, its
not the same as killing someone here, but
there, you do cling to associations and
attachments (Karmic associations), so there
are payments accessed. Whatever you do in
VR can and will create positive and
negative payments to some degree. So the
point here is that once this technology is in
full force, use it wisely. In fact, most are not
aware of it, but when you watch a movie
when fully involved, it carries Karmic
associations unless you detach from it and
few do.

QVRC Relationships

Here we get to the most profound part of
this QVRC technology. It is pretty obvious
that our human relationships are the most
powerful spiritual part of our lives on earth.
Each and every association that you have
with anyone is a spiritual event. Each and
every meeting that you have, no matter how
seemingly unimportant is, is, in fact, an
extremely important spiritual event. You
attitude toward others can never be blown
off with a "Who Cares." Even the most
casual and short association is never an
accident and each occurs as a test to teach
you love. We learn love from every human
51

act. Still our sexual relationships teach us the most and are always key. For a deeper discussion on this, read my book, "Pretty Fine Sex is Spiritual."

QVRC Sex

QVRC will allow each of us to have full mind, body, and voice scans done in labs where you can have them sent and projected anywhere and interactively as you wish and agree. In doing this, anyone can send you their full scans at their discretion sexually or otherwise. They will be able to put a time frame on them or give you permanent files, again at their discretion. Also, anything that you do interactively can be saved and replayed in what amounts to be a real-life movie. Of course, there will be karmic repercussions and much more so than with movies that you just watch. In these, you will live them with no separation.

With this, the bottom line is that you simply agree with someone else and have your virtual person projected interactively or you download them and relate with them if they agree.

QVRC Mentally

So how it works: During the above interaction, once a certain level of
52

information is downloaded into your mental body, your mind becomes saturated and all boundaries are breached. Thus, this is the key to true QVRC power. You simply will not be able to separate the VR experience from your other life experiences, all boundaries will disappear, and you will be there as far as you can detect. With QVRC, when you are in China on a business trip, sex with your wife will be as real as at home, The limits here will go well beyond anything imaginable today and they will far exceed just becoming totally engrossed. Virtually all social barriers will dissolve or take on new meanings since all of the previous warnings regarding sex such as disease and pregnancy will no longer be applicable. With QVRC, our current concerns and our reasons for our current social boundaries will collapse in a heap. Therefore, if you just like someone, you can choose to have sex with them if they agree to exchange their VR files with you. With this degree of openness and interaction, finding a perfect mate should never be a question, but more on this below.

This new level of social freedom, of course, will open up plenty of questions that simple have never arisen in the past, and age differentials will be one of them among the many others. Will we allow kids to again relate to each other as they commonly did in tribal settings and I discuss in "Pretty Fine Sex is Spiritual?" The list will go on as our artificial barriers are breached on a daily basis. How will this affect marriages and our religious concepts. Obviously, this will open the door for almost every social concern ever conceived to be lifted or changed.

Finding the Perfect Mate

The next question is with VR dating: With none of the previous barriers, can we then always find perfect matches? If you look at tribal relationships, prior to current established religious ethics, there may be some applicable answers. However, today, dating entails social games and most everyone plays them to some degree, especially in later adolescence. A few have always breached social barriers and have gone off the supposed deep end, but especially many females have avoided sex out of fears that society, on purpose, imposes.

These fears have often been very effective till at maybe age 21 or thereabouts, when some discover that they have made a terrible mistake. But with QVRC, these often outright lies should never occur again and make no obvious sense. So after many virtual adventures and mistakes, by the time you pick a mate, you should absolutely
54

know exactly what you want in them... then
you have kids and not before. Essentially,
the Annunaki never divorce for this reason,
They have been there and done that far too
many times to need to look further. There
may be no guarantees, but this is very close.
Its especially important to have a nearly
perfect mate when you are apt to live several
thousand years. Living in an imperfect
relationship for sixty years is enough of a
problem, but you need to be close to
perfection to go thousands of years with the
same mate.

Annunaki

Breeding

https://www.youtube.com/watch?v=kQsy
4cM09bQ
The Annunaki/ the gene splicing and cloning
people

https://www.youtube.com/watch?v=GtLh
ENMsdNs *(35)*
The late Lloyd Pye above teaches us more
about the Annunaki

Because of Annunaki breeding, we have a
few genetic disorders that I will point out
that can be controlled easily with
epigenetics, such as our inability to
manufacture Vitamin C. However, we
55

mainly are set up to live eight hundred or
many more years if we play out our
Annunachi cards that are absolutely
contained in your deck of genes. Your
genes are your pliable body blue prints. The
fact is that prior to the Annunachi
inbreeding we were in many ways just like
all other animals with no general systematic
problems and a very robust biology, but
limited to relatively short life spans, and less
aware and intelligent in many ways.

So the Cro Magnon/ Annunaki with their
superior social skills, spirituality and
intelligence won the day in Europe after
they left Mesopotamia/ Sumaria, But the
Annunaki somewhat outfoxed themselves as
they attempted to breed a superior group of
people to mine their gold.   The following
video is absolutely mainstream history, yet
the time frames are obviously subject to
dispute, given the most recent discoveries.
Scan it as it is worth a quick glance:

https://video.search.yahoo.com/yhs/search
?fr=yhs-pty-pty_email&hsimp=yhs-
pty_email&hspart=pty&p=youtube+cro+
magnon+man#id=3&vid=42dbce69dd4f27
b553925ed2ec9de3e3&action=view
Neanderthal v Cro Magnon: this above
video conflicts quite a bit with what the first
two videos. It assumes that neither were

capable of modern human speech abilities. So this video is well produced, but just as likely pure speculation based on unproven theories. In fact, it is just as likely that Neanderthals are with us today as modern humans and did not go anywhere.

Breeding Disorders

Now for ways of dealing with the common disorders and there are a few. Commonly, most animals in the wild are very tough and do not contract the various semi-inherited diseases that are common in society today. Almost all can be reversed with the various supplements outlined in "It's the Liver Stupid" 5th edition, certainly, DMSO and MSM will eliminate most of them. Especially effective is to combine any clean, organic supplements with DMSO. An example would be to take DMSO mixed with D3, P5P (B6), B-12 MCB, and Taurine. I recommend at least 2 tablespoons of MSM swished with water per day for anyone over fifty, but much more for eighty year olds once they have acclimated to taking it.

With the above, the result of our breeding mistakes can be overridden. When you combine this with epigenetics you can basically override all of them, making you essentially equal to the
57

Annunachi. Thus as an equal, you too can live thousands of years. Now listen to this long term DMSO/ MSM expert Bill Rich who has an experience equal to mine in most respects. Below he documents what I have taught and written about, but he does not know the underlying mechanism methylation cycles but is aware far beyond the common knowledge of these two oxygen transport chemicals. MSM/DMSO is in fact a quantum healer that begins at the mitochondrial level as my books teach:

https://www.youtube.com/watch?v=xGh8XeWclIU

The bottom line is that DMSO is the most powerful oxidant (which kill germs by burning them up) on earth and MSM is most powerful antioxidant on earth (which scavenge free radicals that cause aging) and the two transport interactively within the body four or more times when either is ingested. Both work interactively with most any supplement as well as any vitamin, especially C, D, B, E, calcium, magnesium and virtually anything it meets in your body whether stored or ingested. Everything Bill Rich reports on here is correct. He is the most knowledgeable reporter that I have seen on this oxygen transport pair that I first discovered in about 1996.

I had never found that it protects against poisonous snake bites and I do not plan to test it on mambas, but I am certainly not affected by wasps and mosquitoes. After about three years on these two, you do not ever get become ill, period. I have taken as much as 1/2 cup per day of MSM in divided doses when I was hurting with arthritis and joint problems. Furthermore, if you missed exercising and you are stiff, take some extra and it will loosen you up strangely enough just as if you did not.

Now if all of the above is true, what can kill you? An accident? Sure, but these are the basic chemicals behind the ART, now let's live like the Annunachi. As Bill says, it is all about cause.

Who Were the Inbred?

So who were the Cro Magnon really? We know from clay tablets that the Annunaki absolutely inbred with some ancient hominoid groups. Were they Cro Magnon, the result of a Neanderthal Annunaki cross or was there a Cro Magnon/ Annunaki injection that resulted in a superior group of Cro Magnons? So the enlightened Cro Magnon in this story may be Neanderthal/ Annunachi cross of nearly 30k BC (pre-flood) and this assumed Neanderthal/ Cro-

59

Magnon clash may well be an illusion of science that actually never occurred.

This theories of Charles Darwin may be quite different than what he conceived. The genetic model may work very differently than science accepts and I suggest herein. Listen to Dr. Bruce Lipton's idea on genetics and it influence on your life and pay attention to how you actually influence your genetic code subconsciously through epigenetics. This is a game changer, no matter how you resolve it. This puts any defective genes inherited from this Annunaki inbreeding squarely back in your hands and any mistakes well within your discretion.

https://www.youtube.com/watch?v=vDmosJI6b2Q

The above story may be well documented on the Sumerian clay tablets that have yet to be read. Certainly, it can all be interpreted from what is already deciphered.   There is no real evidence that Neaderthal's were/are less intelligent than anyone alive today, especially when you inject Annunaki genomes into them. Furthermore, the Cro Magnon may just be a separate line of people and not basic to our hominoid stock.
60

Imagine that it is 4million years ago, they were likely on earth then and remain on earth as people today. This all, in fact, it dowses as true for me and I have known a few very intelligent people with Neanderthal features, yet their children did not look like them. Their offspring look very much like modern man.

My first book, now in its fifth edition, "It's the Liver Stupid," gives you the supplements and tricks to help you weather these social storm waged against us. You must understand them to make the leaps discussed herein. Going back though, I give you the things to avoid that were not the really the point of those books, which pointed out the building blocks of health, the supplements, and how to use them, but prepare you for the many social aspects that followed including one: the advent of a very long existence. With each passing day, there are some new discoveries as we move forward toward this new paradigm at a pace never seen or remotely anticipated in recent times as Quantum Science begins to displace those same obviously inaccurate and now mostly discredited Newtonian beliefs that must be abandoned as we move into enlightened science. Indeed, Quantum Science is a science by any measure, but especially when you reduce the definition to being able to predict outcomes reputably. But if you
61

are waiting for a current Newtonian science breakthrough to save you, You are going to die waiting. It will not come and cannot possibly occur.

Changes in the Scientific Community

I find it interesting after twenty years of practicing and studying this quantum science (actually twice that before I knew the term), the web is full of newly transformed experts. The Newtonians that have seen see the light to some degree. They are educated firmly in the old science and they carry plenty of credentials as they now see the error in their ways and come across slowly. They miss many of the key points, yet they still have the floor and hold the microphone as PhD's, so they now consider themselves as experts in Quantum Science. However, notice that they often miss the mark in many areas, but they still endorse some of the new findings as they struggle with these new obvious facts that make no sense to them. They will not truly understand the nuances till they get the whole picture. So, consider this when you listen to them speak... use care in listening to their premises which are often flawed. The may have PhD's in Newtonian Science, but these rules violate everything that they were taught and just do not correlate, so they

no longer hold. These indoctrinated aspects
are difficult to give up.

All of my books are full of web references,
mostly You Tube videos here, but some
books also. Mostly, these are the firmly
entrenched experts with Quantum Healing/
QH background that allows them to hold the
microphone and teach you the ropes, but
also there are a few new people who are
excited and suddenly awakened and some
mainstream who serve up long observed
facts to prove my points such as the Key
Ted Lecture below.

Sound, the Primal Source

Lets begin by establishing what must always
be keep in mind and where you place your
attention, Sound. Sound is the primal source
of all vibration and vibration creates light.
Light is the first energy source that religions
recognize because they lack the awareness
to know this.

https://video.search.yahoo.com/yhs/search
?fr=yhs-pty-pty_email&hsimp=yhs-
pty_email&hspart=pty&p=youtube+annu
naki+and+ancient+hidden+tec

The Annunachi taught this and it is true.
Listen for this sound in your head and place
your attention on it. As you do, the sound

63

will increase in volume and value and it will
attract the light. This alone will help keep
you young. Attention, Consciousness, and
Awareness equal unattached love   More on
that below, but listen to this first:
https://video.search.yahoo.com/yhs/search
?fr=yhs-pty-pty_email&hsimp=yhs-
pty_email&hspart=pty&p=You+Tube+Ja
mes+Robert+Clark+Quantum#id

Realize that all disease is a result of low
vibrations and vibrations are born in sound.
Sound vibrations produce light and colors,
A rainbow begins with sound vibrations and
you are a result of sound. This first video
deals with Cancer which begins, as it says
with toxins, but there can be many other
influences as it progresses. If you vibratory
rates were never compromised, you would
always be at the top of your game and well,
no matter what your age and this is a key
point of this book . So music is sound and
music can heal. Art is light and art can heal
The voice of a loving person can heal, just
as the voice of a hateful person can make
you sick. But think about it. You already
knew this. The point of this is to simply
remind you of the knowledge that you were
born with and maybe have not considered
recently. Its all there for you to reestablish
and use in this rebirth. There is nothing new
here for you other than the technologies that
64

are reappearing as we bring them back from
Mesopotamia/ Samaria where science was
awakened. .

An Exercise in De-aging

This key element, sound, spiritually is the
key to everything . Now keeping that in
mind, always listen that the sound between
your ears. Now add the following videos
while keeping your ears attuned to that
sound then go here:
**https://www.youtube.com/watch?v=7V0ti
WtouMA**

While the above video is fun, you do not
need video to go to that place within. This
spiritual exercise is always available and the
sound really never disappears. You may not
always hear it, but it is always there to hear.
Putting you attention on it expands your
universe and builds you spiritually. You
have no age really. Time is an illusion, but
as a person on earth, you must to some
degree buy into it.

False Science

Nearly all that we endorse today as fact is
false from science to art. Let's start with the
gospel of Science as it was handed to us by
the Annunachi where science originated.

65

The facts on the Annunachi will be revealed
as what is proven will also come out but this
is a start:
https://video.search.yahoo.com/yhs/search
?fr=yhs-pty-pty_email&hsimp=yhs-
pty_email&hspart=pty&p=You+Tube+Ja
mes+Robert+Clark+Quantum#id=14&vi
d=f727dba606a5dd482bd63509dbcd673a
&action=view

People, whether they are scientists or
cobblers hate change. Scientists will ague
that they are cutting edge and that they are
reporting exactly what they have discovered.
Some are more direct and honest than others
and their reporting organizations will claim
equal objectivity. with the following videos,
I prove that this is hogwash as the facts are
often set aside or worse so as to maintain the
status quo. These are long videos, but I will
outline the findings and conclusions of the
reporting scientists. To know that I am
correct watch them, but what we as a world
agree to is astounding compared to the
actual conclusive facts and the topic can
range from plants to Darwinian evolution to
planets... what we consider established fact,
religion aside. Herein, I give you just a few,
but you will get the idea. If you have not
seen it yourself, it is often an illusion.
Some of this, you could set aside as garbage
till you hear and see everything as the events
of 911 to the time man has been on earth.
66

These are established scientists who have absolute proofs set aside in favor of status quo.

So you ask, what does this have to do with Anti-aging and De-aging? You have been lied to about virtually every facet of your life. You have been sold on the fact that your paper money has value. That drugs extend your life. That man is very new to the planet, but evolved from apes. And the lies get deeper as the curious and real experts delve into the facts, but little of what we are taught in school has any merit at all. With the Quantum World, as we learn without any possibility of contradiction, all Quantum Mechanical experiments have proven 100% correct to the dismay of Newtonians, while Newtonians are not even close to this level of proof. Now watch this:

Increasing Cognition

These videos tell us, often indirectly, that we can expect increases in mental function through diet since we know that we can increase these blood factors with MSM/ DMSO. So you can expect increases in memory tests and other mental improvements along with reversed physical aging even without our attention on the spiritual aspects:

67

Growing New Neurons

Below we see some of the well know foods
and supplements add to Neurons. Now
adding MSM/DMSO multiplies this factor
many times. Read "It's the Liver Stupid" to
find the many other supplements that are left
out here, but be sure to avoid sugar,
transfats, and toxins per that book.

What to Avoid

The Five Most Dangerous Supplements
While drugs and those who recommend
them are mostly to be avoided, there are a
few examples of them that actually do have
benefits. Obviously, since drugs are about
profits, you are not going to hear many
advertisements for them that go beyond
FDA requirements and the idea that they are

68

required to report on their reactions.
Conversely, Quantum Science is immediate
and transparent. It is not a belief system and
there are no downsides other than social
adjustments, but it does rely on your
accepting it as real, which goes into attitude
and the subconscious that Dr. Bruce Lipton
teaches.

So we think of supplements as avoiding the pitfalls and dangers of these toxins and drugs that control our population today. Below is a report on how these can adversely affect you also:

Mike Adams, the Health Ranger, gives you a wonderful report here: **https://www.youtube.com/watch?v=mFO dLaH2EeMI** I offer this not only because I love what Mike does, but for what he discusses off-hand here. Note that he mentions that Sulfur is a great detoxing agent as it is. Now recall that MSM/ DMSO is probably the greatest detoxing agent on earth as I have reported from many sources in my earlier books. Both give up and receive oxygen molecules as they work and are thus equal in their net effects. The difference is that DMSO does it immediately. So if you need fast relief, delivered topically, this is where you should start. This is only part of that story, but Mike is offering that part correctly. With so much new information on the web, it is impossible to get it all from one source. you have to learn to pick and chose and I suggest that Mike is a good, responsible start.

Second, Mike, off-hand, mentions that
Cacao can contain a good deal of lead.
Cacao is probably the best natural source of
Magnesium on earth, but we have to be
careful with our sources.

Finally, his report agrees with my sources
and my first book that I just updated with
the 5th edition. Listen to Mike. He is telling
you just how it is. MD's and scientists are
just not versed on this level of healing yet
and as Mike advises, your best choice is an
informed naturopath who is a nutritionist.
Still, you have the final say and your body is
mostly unique, treat it wisely and you will
receive the benefits long term... our interest
here.

My interest here is to teach you how to live
as the Annunachi do... eight hundred years
minimum, which is really a child in
Annunachi lifetimes still *(23).*
https://www.youtube.com/watch?v=GtUN
bY7REvI
We are discussing thousands of years here,
really, and you have the key.

71

Some have lived many more, but we are discussing average lifespans, If you are looking to double the normal lifespan or more, you simply cannot be doing what the ignorant uniformed (or government informed) people are doing. When you no longer ingest poisons at a rate higher than your body can expel, and if you are careful, your wonderful systems can do that, you can begin this antiaging/ de-aging journey.

Aging Defined

The Key to This Book

What is aging then? As discussed, you have been told and trained that you must age and that your chronological ages must correlate we those who match your age. Even the speaker in the video below buys into this 20,000 year old paradigm, but he also gets that you are actually better than at any age previously. He, as he says, is not the first or the only expert to come to this conclusion. But you must rise above these social, mental and physical pitfalls before you can truly benefit from the fact that you have survived the negatives of yo9uth as discussed below:

The Mental Part

Listen to this TED Talk carefully, paying attention to his "crystallized processing" discussion and what this expert tells you that growing older does to add to this process. This is really the key aspect of my premise here for this book. But this TED lecture came after my premises was well established. Keep in mind that in science, something that is crystallized is frozen and anything fluid can move: Few understand the quantum aspects of crystals that I report in my earlier books and drive computers. https://www.youtube.com/watch?v=wrTI S0uKg6o

A part of my contribution here is that we can add to the described "fluid processing" and no age deterioration is required or occurs if you follow what I offer. Again, listen to his TED explanation carefully. Aging is a transformation as the speaker says, not a deterioration, in terms of mental activity. This is the premise here. The key, again, is that de-aging is also a transformation and is a subconscious shift in awareness. If your mind is frozen, nothing can occur, So this de-aging process is about total mental and physical flexibility   This action occurs though epigenetics and it is a very natural transformation if you are physically well and on top of your game.

73

There is a degree of protection here. You subconscious needs to know that you can handle it before it will give you the ball. Further, you must convince your subconscious body that you are actually getting younger and you do this with the spiritual exercises. These train your subconscious mind to accept that you are de-aging. When you hear others lost in the aging process talk, realize that they are stuck, frozen both mentally and physically. It is very unlikely that anything that you tell them will breach this subconscious wall that society has built for them.

The Physical Part

This is really the simple part of the puzzle
even though science today sees it as
impossible. This is true because your body
is already on top of this game if it supplied
with the tools it needs. It knows what you
are supposed to be like from the blue print.
The blue print, as Dr. Bruce Lipton tells you
tells it what you are supposed to look like.
It is the Genetic Code in the form of DNA.
As most everyone is aware by now, you
were born with this blue print. What they
seldom know yet is that you, as the architect
of your body, can freely modify the code at
any time through this epigenetics process as
long as you supply the construction
materials to it for the repairs that allow it.
Herein, I tell you how and in my first book,
"It's the Liver Stupid," I give you most of
the specifications for that work, especially
with the fifth edition. The construction may
be completed immediately for minor repairs,
but the period seldom lasts over six months
for most any problem as long as there is a
timely delivery of materials.

In my case, where mistakes were encoded during my mother's first trimester of pregnancy, the above process took longer, but it was obviously underway from its conception and my unconscious mind was well aware that this body was undergoing a total makeover. However, few projects require this degree of transformation and sprit is 100% efficient.

Anti-aging and De-aging ART

So how could a seventy-five year old man know that the above process is even possible and how does it work? Let's begin with some background:

First off, this and all lifetimes are experiments and projects in the works at various levels. Furthermore, we are all subject to and endure traumatic deaths from car collisions, falls, etc. just to keep us on our toes spiritually. Notice that I did not use the word accident, because spirit is, as I said, completely efficient. There really are never any accidents. Furthermore, all deaths are illusions and time, as we know it, is also. Your body always carries an up-to-date blue print set to refer to, but that changes with each lifetime to fit our needs as we progress.

In this world, your mind strays in this
process and is really subject to reversals or
illusions. As it is much like a child. The
higher self that resides in your spiritual aura
must step back and. visualize who you really
are and toss out the conflicts any unruly
conflicts that the child allows to creep in.
Use the spiritual exercises that I offer to aid
to resolve this (also in my other books0.
Certainly, if you attempt to force anything,
you will just increase the problem.
Visualization is always the key, not force.
An unruly mind hates being told forcefully
what to do just a child does. Given the above
premises, it really does not matter whether
you live eight hundred years or die in the
next hour, because you have a spiritual bar
to cross and you will get there no matter
how long it takes or where your unruly mind
may lead you astray. Moreover, if your
mind kills your body off by some means,
memory of this lifetime will generally be
suppressed, next lifetime, and you will
apparently have to start over, but this is
never the case as it is again, 100% efficient
in fact.

Once you achieve the fifth level spiritually, this apparent dark and gloomy repetition basically stops. Then you take control of the situation entirely, releasing yourself from what eastern religions describe as the Wheel of the 84 or Karma. Once you rise to this level of awareness, you can actually chose to came back as you are now the master of your awareness. When you reach this 5th level and choose to be born, you either come here in full awareness or that level of awareness comes back to you quickly and you have a free hand to make your spiritual contribution. Beyond the 5th, you are basically working as a representative of God and that has to be where your attention is placed.

There are ways of reconstructing past life memories, but even doing that generally entails living a longer than normal lifetime, Even though most children carry some previous life memory till about age five when they mostly abandon them as illusion. If you disagree, ask these younger kids questions about their previous lives. You may be shocked, but they will accept your questions openly, without fanfare, and generally take them seriously. But their comments will blow you away if you give them your full attention and they will love you for it, since they get few chances, if any, to tell of them to real listeners.

78

The interest here is to get you back to where
you were prior to being five years old, so to
speak, then growing your wisdom and
spirituality from there. A good portion of
the population over seventy and certainly
over eighty today suffers from conscious
memory loss of even this lifetime, let alone
past lives. Furthermore, their sight and
hearing, but even taste and feel have
declined. None of these losses are necessary
or even genetically programmed in as we are
led to believe. Even if you must wear
glasses today and you require a hearing aid,
it is not so difficult to recover these senses.
Without them, you will obviously miss a
great deal and, in fact, the youth may just
may even try to avoid you.

A good part of gathering wisdom and spirituality is so that you can pass this insight and knowledge on to the youth especially (but maybe a few others, generally). After all, you have been enduring the hardships of life at fifteen, even maybe at twenty times the level that they have seen thus far   Kids may be well aware of previous lives, certainly, but what they do not have available consciously is the wisdom that they gathered in those past lives. It really takes seventy or eighty years to pull this together. Furthermore, given that few today live longer than that, our actual gains per lifetime are relatively very low. Further, if you manage to live a few hundred years, think about it, how much more will you acquire? The United States has only been around two-hundred and forty two years as of this writing. What if you could relate what really happened at the signing of the Magna Carta or Napoleon's invasion or even the Civil War? We know that yesterday's news and history is seldom close to accurate, but you could put it all in context. You would become a new shining light of wisdom. Herein, I am suggesting that this is a real possibility, given the Quantum Biology that is coming into view together with the abandonment of drugs and disease.

80

So how do we get this done? Quite possibly, I have lost credibility here with many Newtonian based scientists, but please try to stay with me as I point out proofs based on ancient Sumerian tablets, existing built structures, and, again, Quantum Science. Taken as a whole, these are overwhelming proof that you are indeed, part Annunachi and you hold within you, the biology that can allow you at least another three hundred years of wisdom. Obviously, no one in the last thousand years carried this wisdom with them.

During the dark ages, people lived much shorter periods than even today and in the past two thousand years most likely lived half our average life span even today. In ancient Scotland, burial sites suggest that you had maybe twenty years to complete the entire life process on average and the very oldest were maybe fifty years old. We could go on as to why, but the point here is that we can go back to what the leaders were doing pre-flood in Samaria. The Christian Bible states that they were living eight hundred years or so. Rumanian clay tablets tell you that their leaders lived much longer. In fact, some may have lived two-thousand years.

So, you say, who wants to live two
thousand years (and. I ask you what would
your knowledge base be if you were on the
Council of Nicea as they discussed who
Jesus really was? What could you add to
this discussion? What would life be like for
those who heard you?

Teaching Your Mind

Back to Dr. Bruce Lipton's epigenetics, the
subconscious education,
https://www.youtube.com/watch?v=mNT
UwIFslKM

https://www.youtube.com/watch?v=HnF
Cz6UCakk   Newton Physics explained *(9)*
Dogma *(12)* Genetic Determinism *(12.55)*
Causes of Death*(14.20)*

I notice that today, Bruce is aging at a rather
normal rate (and jokes/ admits it in the 2nd
video above) since he first became that
headliner speaker that he is, not to discredit
Bruce. He is absolutely correct in what he
teaches for the most part, but he is would
have stopped aging if he had had the full
story and even gotten younger in the last ten
years. Nevertheless, listen to what he is
teaching here on a paradigm shift.

82

Consciousness, which is awareness of who you are and all that you encounter, is a key element in spirituality. By the way, consciousness is unlimited and you can never fill up your head with too much information as he suggests here at first. In fact, your mind does not reside in your head as he first suggests. So the bottom line is that consciousness simply does not reside there, But yes, you do gain when you share awareness and this is where you as a spiritual being gain more in consciousness awareness. In fact, there is no limit to anything spiritual and these are absolutely elements of spirituality.

Wisdom does not equal awareness, but it absolutely grows with consciousness and experience key contributors to wisdom if you are aware. One of the key elements to aging then is wisdom and wisdom can be passed on to any aware people who are paying attention. You can be aware and still focusing on other things, so these are not identical attributes.

By the way, listening to Bruce, and you can
check me out on any of my facts with
dowsing, fish will not be dead in thirty
years, and his answers, wind power and
solar panels will not save this planet and in
fact are inferior examples of energy saving
solutions at least as they are employed
today. We must keep our attention on the
Quantum Science which can change such
conclusions dramatically.

My point at the beginning here is that people
like Mike Adams and Dr. Bruce Lipton have
many of the answers, but as a reporter, my
interest is to place your attention on various
pieces of the solution. Mike has a
laboratory that examines the foods and
supplements that we eat. Bruce has put his
attention on proving that genetics were
incorrectly given too much credit and that
we can rise above the genetic profiles that
we were given us by the Annunachi prior to
the flood.

We must gain wisdom to make this system
work and Bruce is correct that stress must be
let go of and dropped. You will not De-age
if stress is controlling your life. Now listen
carefully to what he says about Quantum
Science, Spirit, and Awareness. The city
that he discusses was governed by the
Annunachi.
**https://video.search.yahoo.com/yhs/search
?fr=yhs-pty-pty_email&hsimp=yhs-
pty_email&hspart=pty&p=You+Tube+Ja
mes+Robert+Clark+CP4U#id=2&vid=c3
96a384d6ec2aa388ad57ced4dee70a&actio
n=view** This is the Mesopotamia of the
bible.
**https://www.youtube.com/watch?v=3TIc
VJGfjLU**

Old Testament Bible

The old testament (OT) is a rewriting of the thousands Sumarian/ Mesopotamian clay tablets. There is nothing in the OT that was not a rewriting of their history. While the Sumarian tablets were essentially etched in stone, the OT was written on parchment paper and much of it was lost. The Sumerians knew that with fired clay, as most of their world died off, there would be no loss and it would survive. You can buy eight thousand year old Sumarian clay tablets online, by the way and they are as readable as the day they were fired while the Dead Sea Scrolls are mostly lost even though they are likely all redundant.

Despite Bruce's concerns, ocean fish will survive and people will not go the way of dinosaurs.
Check for yourself, but things can change. A nuclear war would change this outcome for instance. Also, Bruce contradicts himself with his earlier observation as he reports that an EEG is not about consciousness just as he reports. Magneto encephalographs do not measure consciousness either, but he is correct here that the mind is a receiver and this is all stored outside your head in the field.

Growing Young Gracefully

Quantum Magic is not magic at all, but this is the Quantum Biology (QB) that will allow you to transcend the biology that mainly controls our population today. Now watch this as Richard Gordon reports on what Dr. Richard Price and I have been reporting on this for some thirty or more years and Paul Twitchell was telling us in the 1960's:
https://www.youtube.com/watch?v=M8FF6j4Kcco&t=55s
"The Secret Nature of Matter," Richard Gordon This stuff absolutely rubs off as Richard says.
Water All matter is God stuff. Correctly guessing (?) as we do using dowsing. Now take what Richard is discussing which is mainly alignment. There is no disease or condition that cannot be healed. This my friend Dr. Price and I have proven. Still what Richard Gordon has found is absolutely correct. Now realize that his pendants are not as strong as the lab crystals that we use today and have used on cars. These Quantum healing devices heal machines (Quantum Mechanics) just as well as they heal people (Quantum Biology) and make plants grow at astounding rates:
https://video.search.yahoo.com/yhs/search?fr=yhs-pty-pty_email&hsimp=yhs-pty_email&hspart=pty&p=You+Tube+James+Robert+Clark+CP4U#id=1&

Social Adjustments

Nothing can prepare you for what this book can deliver if you follow it carefully and with passion. I discussed it to some degree in my book, "Pretty Fine Sex is Spiritual," and even to a smaller degree in "It's the Liver Stupid," but here as the targeted audience is older, with more wisdom and hopefully now using both sides of their minds, with this, the social aspects become even more profound if you have learned to avoid the pitfalls that aging can bring. First, there is no getting around the fact that society expects you to follow what is normal and die at age 80 or thereabouts. for the rare few who live to be 100, they will insist that you go into a home for the aged even if your cellular age is that of a 16 year old and you are mentally clear as a bell with full use of your mind, something that you never previously had.

Obviously, our government is not prepared for what we will be and already, I am continually offered classes on hearing aids, etc. even though my hearing is awesome as is my vision. More on that below.

88

Society will likely take hundreds of years to adjust to what you attain and you cannot wait for them to catch up. They are certain that life belongs to the youth, while the facts do not bear this out.

Avoiding Toxins

Toxins are a part of natures systems, but herein, I give you ways to circumvent them for the most part. At one extreme, sun gazing as we see can make you into what is known as a God Eater, allowing you to avoid food entirely and completely avoid eating toxins completely and that is your primary source of then. However, they can be breathed or absorbed through the skin or more likely, for most of us, be induced from things sold as healthy such as beauty aids and even supposedly curative drug carriers. Even commercial products sold to cover up body odor, deodorants, generally are somewhat toxic. But in today's society you are surrounded by toxins and even in ancient times they were prevalent in nature. The Romans used perfumes and deodorants for this reason and they still do.

Smell and Body Odor

As people age in our present society, our senses
diminish and this, today, this is accepted as a
normal part of aging, but the only part of aging
that we accept in this book's premise is that we
gain wisdom. But please consider some of these
obviously flawed "facts" that our society and
medical establishment accepts as normal when it
comes to smell as walk you through some
obvious facts that are mostly never considered as
related or in any way associated to each other:

BO is the body freeing itself of toxins, no
matter where they occur as it fights to survive.
We associate races and nationalities with body
smells. Why? Mostly because different cultures
eat different foods and foods, as noted
previously contain various toxins, some of these
may be of little importance to your overall
health and, yes, your body is able to deal with
them, at least on a fifty or hundred year basis
which, again, we commonly accept as a normal
lifetime.

Let's consider some common infections that create smells: Kidney and Bladder infections commonly create urine that smells bad due to bacteria overgrowths. This is associated with invasive bacteria that are creating the infection and in fact, even prior to the body reacting to them, you are warned that smelly urine is a warning sign. In fact, if you had no toxins in your body or very low levels or bacteria overgrowths, your urine would have no odor at all and neither would your feces. It is commonly reported that people with cancer often smell really badly. Why? Cancer is a disease of toxic overload. So a person with cancer is attempting to reject the overload in any way possible and to survive.

Older people often have body odor. Listen to care giver's reports, but why? They have stored up toxins for eighty or ninety years and their bodies must rid themselves of overloads as much as possible to survive. Their underarms, then, smell and their urine and feces will be particularly odorous in many people. We have grown to expect most older people to stink and the warning we give them is to make sure they stay clean. Fortunately, for them, they have a reduced sense of taste and smell, so they are not so affected as the care givers.
People who have had their gall bladders removed have particularly bad smelling feces for the same above reasons. Your gall bladder is an organ that is designed to help free your body of toxins... is this making sense at all?

91

Even the very young in our society have issues associated with their habits and foods. Young girls typically have vaginal odors. Vaginas are just one place that can and do accumulate bacteria and toxins so this is expected. The solution is not for them to douche, but to clean up their eating habits... no sugars, breads, pizza, or MacDonalds and this will not occur. The old addend, you are what you eat is expressed in "you are how you smell." No part of a truly healthy body has a inherent odor in itself.

Particularly deodorants which cover up smells and even worse antiperspirants which commonly use aluminum salts as gels to literally block your sweat glands from functioning, this keep your natural method of freeing toxins and adjusting from even functioning. But the bottom line here is that you should be odor free with no interventions if you are listening. This is just another huge industry that should fail along with sunscreens and blocks and they even sound similar.

http://www.antiperspirantsinfo.com/en/

Why Our Systems Fail

There is a common and overriding theme
and it currently is age related. Here is why:
you were born with a fair amount of
nutrients if you were lucky. They have
everything to do with what you scavenged
from your mother during pregnancy. During
gestation, you were number one, but if she
lacked nutrients, you both failed. The first
trimester was the most critical when you
were evolving with rapid cell division. If she
missed something during this critical event
in growth, you will carry that error unless
you can make it up with large amounts later
and that is difficult.

So in my case, I had what is known as
juvenile arthritis. This is cased by a critical
lack of sulfur then. I took this deficiency
into my forties. It included a hip joint
problem, migraines, and fingers swelling
when cold. With knowledge of MSM at very
high levels, these problem subsided and no
longer occur.

Interestingly, my mother grew up on a farm and ate pretty well, but somewhere she missed. For her, this meant horrible lower back pain for her entire life. This problem was mostly prevalent with her nine siblings also. One or two did not suffer with this ailment. If you asked an MD, the answer would be that they all inherited the same genetic predisposition to lower back problems. Listen to what Dr. Bruce Lipton teaches about genes, but in nearly every case, all health conditions have a basis in diet. The best explanation is that my grandmother lacked the nutrients in her diet during the first trimester and passed on these traits. If this were not the case, I would have died of a heart condition where I was headed.

With all of these joint ailments, when I entered my thirties, my arms and legs would commonly "go to sleep." I thought this was normal and often, my friends complained of the same condition. They have all since died of heart attacks. I have no friends alive today that I grew up with. A few died of cancer as most of my mother's siblings did. But this is a very different condition, for a long discussion on cancer, read, "Between the Jeans," my last book.

So, there is a common theme with all of the conditions below. When any of your senses begins to fail, it is invariably about a lack of flexibility and tissue hardening, so can be relieved with DMSO/ MSM either directly applied or through ingestion, but also this can be ameliorated with proper dietary nutrients. Certainly, correct amounts of MSM will put your body back into Annunaki genetic territory if done very long.

While you are commonly taught otherwise, our senses do not go away with age and sex, when you are on your game should be at least a daily event. Prostate problems for men should never occur and there should be no such thing as a change of life for women. If there is a lack of hormones, it is because something is hardening and is not your penis. So it is all tissue failure and if is the joints often, where it shows up first. The lack of tissue compliance or resiliency is the main issue as we no longer feed our bodies the correct foods. So read these specific areas below but notice the common cure. Yes, MSM/DMSO do supply a healthy amount of Sulfur, but this is just not the cure alone:

Skin Care

95

As you might guess and certainly the beauty
agents promoted know, creams do soften to
a degree, but at a price as most of them
contain ingredients that are to some degree
actually toxins. I outline those in, "It's the Liver
Stupid" in depth, but the key here is to read
labels and stick to natural ingredients like
coconut oil and aloe vera where you are mostly
safe.

Skin, as the commercials tell you, is a question
of softness and lifts are a temporary but short
term approach to what DMSO will permanently
cure. This, especially if you are complementing
it with MSM in your diet as you should be. But
when you find something that is effective, add
DMSO to it and it will multiply the system.

Eye Care

My sight at age 18 was 20/50 ns today I can
read the bottom line on a sight chart with
either eye, but my eyes will tire and I do use
1.5 cheaters in bad light when they do, but I
am working on that. Now realize that at age
50, I was using 3.5 magnifiers and could
not read small print without them, but that
was prior to taking high level MSM on a
daily basis. Relax your eyes and do not
stare, glance away and let them work for
you, now lets discuss why and how you can
ditch glasses at any age, but mainly about
magnifiers which stop your eyes from
learning:

Sun Gazing Exercises that have shown
benefits and give us D3 which has eye (plus
many other) benefits. Scan these videos
based on time in doing gazing only at
sunrise and set:

9minutes/day

https://www.youtube.com/watch?v=FN2u
7P1wUQU
1/2 hour/day.   (He is correct on the 90,000
IU part it were at noon)
https://www.youtube.com/watch?v=
WIZpmReB6gU
45 minutes/day
https://www.youtube.com/watch?v=zjf_U
RaDTRY

For 3 hours a day *(3.0)*

The advice on this video follows what we are warned by mainstream, but is unproven https://www/day.youtube.com/watch?v=QLDx5wSXUeE and does not follow my own experience.

My own experience started at age four when my now considered, "ignorant friends," and I would lie down to see just how close we could come to looking directly into the sun. We did this fairly often as I recall. Then, some 20 years ago I met a very intelligent local scientist who recommended doing it again, but only at 12 noon when UV was highest. So by his advice, given today's accepted (and undisputed) science I should be blind! So what did I gain (or lose) from this. First, on the 2nd go around, I noticed that my floaters mainly disappeared and my reading level eyesight improved from needing 3.5 diopter readers to occasional 1.5's when I get tired or under very low light, but I was using MSM/ DMSO starting at about that same time, so it is virtually impossible to separate the reason for my vision improvement.

My question from the above is... has anyone ever proven that UV will harm your eyes even if you look at it directly? Could past safe hours just be another old wives tale? Testimony on the web would seem to bear this out as so, but these are the same idiots that are recommending sunscreen and causing skin cancer. Finally, I never did (do) it till it became very uncomfortable. or less than a few minutes unlike this guy who went a half hour and was temporarily blinded but recovered. This video is more in keeping with my own experience, but it still misses what I do:
https://www.youtube.com/watch?v=iUsU4STxIJc

Hair Loss and Graying

I am not affected by thinning hair, but my readers who are report that their hair is filling back in from just taking high level MSM. Read the chapter, "The Oxygen Transport Pair" as coined by Dr. David Gregg who I dedicated several chapters to in, "It's the Liver Stupid."

So how do you get back graying or white hair to your natural color and no, white is not natural. First, virtually every result that we attribute to aging is about tissue hardening and inflexibility. This DMSO half of the Oxygen Transport Pair can be combined with any virtually any other supplement that compliments them when delivered to the tissue. For hair color or thinning, DMSO when applied directly will aid in hair regrowth and this has been reported by many. They did it by just using MSM orally. Obviously, direct application is more powerful as this is a transdermal treatment and it can deliver far more, more quickly.

Read my first book to know what to avoid in terms of shampoos, etc. as many are just poisons and combining them with DMSO, the most powerful delivery system on earth, is a very bad idea. Still, applying DMSO to your scalp will soften the hair follicles and darken white hair. Now, per Dr. Joel Wallach's animal observations, hair lightens because your follicles are deprived of organic copper, so mix some in the DMSO.

Hearing

My hearing is awesome and by my own tests with my sound system conclude that it is good from 20Hz to 20,000. Thus, it is better than most 16 year olds. The solution to anti-aging is to take High Level MSM orally, which is DMSO. If your hearing has already declined, your solution is to use DMSO eardrops. Topical DMSO is incredibly powerful. The problem with hearing is that your ear drums and components have hardened. You really have no other means of gaining that flexibility back except through direct application into the ear.

Again, read my report as mentioned above in "It's the Liver Stupid" to see how this "Oxygen Transport Pair" works, but this was proposed some ten years ago, after Stanly Jacobs first reported on these two organic chemicals. No one reports or have even attempted to prove this out, but given the results that these yield, this, with the now well established Methyl Pathways are the only explanation as to how DMSO can rescue your hearing, but it is now understood

Joint Care

101

This is where the MSM/ DMSO protocols began. I tell the story in depth in my first book, but its still unbelievably effective in repair any joint problem from back pain to knees. The most common story is: "but I have no other choice other than knee replacement surgery. My knee is bone to bone." The answer is that your body recalls every aspect of good health. It knows what it is supposed to look like and how it should perform. In order to have degraded to this condition, you have kept the necessary repair nutrients from it. Interestingly, if it is missing these nutrients, you are on the path to heart and circulatory disease. Why is this? The veins and arteries are comprised of the same tissue and it is just a matter of time before your circulatory system hardens and your heart can no longer adjust to the fact that there is no longer any compliance in your system. System failure is well on the way. It is inevitable and it is the main cause of death today.

Attitude

Transdermal Solutions

DMSO/ MSM
https://www.youtube.com/watch?v=e8a2m2VO9k0

Cancer Causes
https://www.youtube.com/watch?v=b_D4ng
5Od2A&t=1023s
https://video.search.yahoo.com/yhs/search?f
r=yhs-pty-pty_email&hsimp=yhs-
pty_email&hspart=pty&p=You+tube+james
+robert+Clark+quantum#id=

Sulfur DMSO/**MSM**
**https://video.search.yahoo.com/yhs/search
?fr=yhs-pty-pty_email&hsimp=yhs-
pty_email&hspart=pty&p=You+Tube+Ja
mes+Robert+Clark+CP4U#id=2**
Water Certainly Richard Gordon was
mostly correct as were the others that I
reference herein. However, Gordon had no
Living Water to compare or experiment with

Sound: Much has been written on sound and
today we know that sound is the basis for all
things and it very different as these videos
contend compared to what mainstream
Newtonian science holds as fact.

Monatomic Gold (MG) and Ormes

Today, we can make and buy monatomic
gold online and even make it ourselves, but
this has been documented in ancient
Annunachi texts and much later in OT the
bible, so again it is written in stone (fired
clay) and proven.

This white MG powder is sound/ gold captured as light also termed as Manna in the bible. This MG is no longer a supposition and not just known in biblical times which are relatively recent where this report begins. In fact, it does not even begin with Sumaria/ Mesopotamia. The important thing here is the message that we are just beginning to recapture the lost knowledge that the Annunachi brought here over some 400,000 years ago. The significant key part of the disclosure that is the MG is a part of our anti-de-aging system presented here. The discussion on the video below regarding de-aging is with regard to telomere length, still not totally documented by science, but almost totally likely at least a measure of aging and possibly a piece of the de-aging puzzle.

Ormes can be based on many minerals and each has anti-aging/ de-aging properties. All are valuable and significant including silver, gold, platinum, and other noble metals, but keep in mind that in ormes is captured vibration that does the work and despite what is reported, you as a spiritual being can capture sound and light. Therefore, we carry antigravity spiritually.

 Below is a very general overview on this topic with many historic references:
104

https://www.youtube.com/watch?v=9jw8CI6eyl0

The reference below are more technical an less broad from an author who makes MG:
http://search.hemailaccessonline.com/?uid=72cd844a-6357-43ec-8634-4c0f2a2ed475&uc=20171023&ap=appfocus1&source=googlesearch-googlesearch-v3&page=newtab&implementation_id=email_4.0.17

David Hudson, the guy who discovered Ormes and his discovery:
https://www.youtube.com/watch?v=klbJhwxxqDE

Teleomeres/Telemerase

The mainstream is certain that the telemeres
are the secret to antiaging and to some
degree it is possible, but when you look at
the causes of death as telomere shortening
then you wonder. There is definitely an
association between telomere shortening and
life span though. However, the question is
always what is cause and what is effect in
this relationship and can we increase
shortened teleomers? For example, if you
look at skin wrinkling, you might well
make the same association between wrinkles
and aging. So does skin wrinkling cause
death? If we manage to get rid of wrinkles,
will you live longer? Obviously, unless
your wrinkles go away do to health yes, but
if scientists learn to lengthen telomeres with
drugs, there is almost no chance that you
will live an extra day.

I suggest that this is just another example of
a dog chasing its tale, but sounds great and
people are making huge amounts of money
researching another rainbow of science,
while new these magic bullet concepts are
created that sound wonderful. It will just
never
happen. https://video.search.yahoo.com/yhs/se
arch;_ylt=AwrC5pYWMGlaG3UAI1I0nIlQ;
_ylu=X3oDMTBncGdyMzQ0BHNlYwNzZW
FyY2gEdnRpZANM-
;_ylc=X1MDMTM1MTE5NTcwMARfcgMy
BGFjdG4DY2xrBGJiawM5dTZpdnQ1Y21u
ajc3JTI2YiUzRDQlMjZkJTNEOUw2TGouc
HBZRUtrVkJ6UGgwVkVORXRidTZhMGl
ZMm9VTzNtdnctLSUyNnMlM0RpaSUyNm
klM0RLSmVrRm1rR0daOVRrZlpxZmVxbg
Rjc3JjcHZpZANlbXlnU3pFd0xqR2ZHbF9w
V1d2TTV3a0NNVEE0TGdBQUFBQ0tCVV
Q5BGZyA3locy1wdHktcHR5X2VtYWlsBGZ
yMgNzYS1ncARncHJpZANBYWZma09VS1
JhS0ZlOFV4b01WQ0lBBG10ZXN0aWQDbn
VsbARuX3JzbHQDNjAEbl9zdWdnAzAEb3
JpZ2luA3ZpZGVvLnNlYXJjaC55YWhvby5j
b20EcG9zAzAEcHFzdHlDBHBxc3RybAME
cXN0cmwDMzUEcXVlcnkDeW91dHViZSB0
ZWxvbWVyZXMgYWdpbmcgRXBpZ2VuZ
XRpY3MEdF9zdG1wAzE1MTY4NDM3NTg
EdnRlc3RpZANudWxs?gprid=AaffkOUKRa
KFe8UxoMVCIA&pvid=emygSzEwLjGfGl
pWWvM5wkCMTA4LgAAAACKBUT9&p=
youtube+telomeres+aging+Epigenetics&ei=U
TF-
8&fr2=p%3As%2Cv%3Av%2Cm%3Asa&fr
=yhs-pty-pty_email&hsimp=yhs-

107

In every case, Newtonian science will take the high tech pathway when the question is asked of what causes health and aging.. So here, you will hear that teleomeres are a contributory cause of Aids, Cancer, and Heart disease, among many others. Herein, I suggest that these diseases cause shortened teleomeres, so when you die, the scientists measure them as proof of this flawed premise.

My dowsing also agrees that, as is common, they have their story backward. So the premise reported above is that cancer is caused by genetic defects and the premise here is that cancer is a total body defense system where the body is reacting to toxins and, and as a result, changes its chemistry to save you even if just a short time. Plant extracts that this scientist is experimenting with will never be as effective as foods as whole foods because plants are brilliant combinations of biological chemistry. Basically, plant extracts are one step away from pharmaceutical drugs and they deplete entrained sunlight just as cooking does.

Disease

Dr. Joel Wallach tells us why its always about Epigenetics and Nutrition and not genes:
https://www.youtube.com/watch?v=4K_A yjgPXfg

108

I have followed Wallach since his tape and reported on him extensively in, "Its the Liver Stupid." It is hard to fault his clear logics, intuition, and observations when it comes to human disease, especially as he relates to it to the health o animals.

Hot Tub Reinvented
Ocean Water/ DMSO Solution

The above, Hot Tub/Ocean Water/ DMSO Solution when combined with monatomic gold and other nutrients is the most biologically de-aging combination possible. This is a long-term solution that basically was used to de-age and regress the Annunaki every few hundred years and is still commonly employed by them today. It heals as a transdermal solution, but adding organic supplements to further help a hot tub will entail changing the water as required, but there are huge benefits here over inorganic solutions alone and the technology has never been developed in our era thus far.

But first, lets start with Hot Ocean Water which naturally contains a wealth of minerals and hear what others report:

Now why is this true? Note that most people cannot wait to take a fresh water shower after they swim in the ocean. The ocean is not just salt water. Again, it is full of minerals that come from oceanic springs and deep underwater jets that provide a full complement of minerals, though they are not digested by plants, so are not bioavailable orally. In fact, these are the minerals that life grew out of.

Now realize that anything transdermal is superior to oral intake by many times as there is no digestive loss. Sea salt, again, is produced by underwater jets spewed from the earth and while we may taste the salt in it, this is not the part that we are looking for. Salt water fish will die when the minerals are no longer in the salt water, so it is not just the salt. In your case, you will thrive when you spend at least fifteen minutes a day in a sea water hot tub. Probably the best source of your hot tub water would be from the Great Salt Lake but some more dense source is most desirable. This obvious ocean water is the cheaper, but less healing solution. From here, this is an experiment that I plan to include in my hot tub. Obviously, it will work as planned short term, but I know nothing about maintenance or amounts long term.

Adding DMSO, Monatomic Gold and a careful selection of nutrients plus sunlight for full nutritional effects. It all has huge obvious potential. However any organics need careful consideration when added to the mix and must be monitored carefully.

Sea Water Birthing

Before we get into this, you might ask why is a 70-80 year old reading about birthing? Guess...

111

There is proof that this theory that woman are born with x amount of eggs is wrong or at least flawed to a great degree. https://video.search.yahoo.com/yhs/search?fr=yhs-pty-pty_email&hsimp=yhs-pty_email&hspart=pty&p=You+Tube+menopause+theory#id=1&vid=eb56779e40cb380e259c61138955d0a3&action=click If this is even remotely correct, the idea of a set number of eggs at birth is not true and it has been reported that in some societies women in the seventies and older do give birth. But let's get to my favorite related topic:

https://video.search.yahoo.com/yhs/search?fr=yhs-pty-pty_email&hsimp=yhs-pty_email&hspart=pty&p=youtube+assisted+water+birth+control#id=57&vid=903d76d7444d41607f3d6cc7c5d5387b&action=view

The potential for birthing in a hot tubs is now fairly well known, but has been known and reported in You Tube since it was created, but adding salt water and DMSO, etc, creates something beyond conception.

Breach Birth Story

Now the interesting parts of the above story are:
112

Babies need not be turned around in breach
birthing per common procedure.
Chords are easily unwrapped thus are not
the problem assumed.
So this very cute couple avoided hospital
birthing and the questionable procedures
associated with them, but what about a birth
certificate? Was the baby even born by law?

**https://video.search.yahoo.com/yhs/search
?fr=yhs-pty-pty_email&hsimp=yhs-
pty_email&hspart=pty&p=youtube+unas
sisted+water+birth#id=41&vid=a41dc907
2c3da526f9fc78aa3ad09361&action=view**

While the above story is very sweet and
avoids the procedures, it the baby were born
in a salt water hot tub, the transition to
breathing air would be less dramatic and it
would be even move loving. How nice for a
newborn to lay on its mothers breasts rather
than being slapped by a doctor, a procedure
now being abandoned by many.

DMSO

https://www.youtube.com/watch?v=oMtd2g
kxKjg
https://www.youtube.com/watch?v=PoP-
5lnydzA Amanda Dawn Voillmer is new to
DMSO, but she gets how powerful DMSO
is for healing in her short time with it. She
also gets that it is likely the most powerful
oxidant and oxidant delivery healing system
on earth (since it is so well absorbed through
your skin as well as internally). So here is
how you use it in your hot tub: Add at least
1% to your water for the full benefit and, to
get that, you should fully immerse several
times with your eyes open.

I use 100% on my eye lids since it goes right
through them and into my eyes. Plus, I use it
on my face mixed with astaxanthin and
herbs. This, after a shower when the pores
are open and every day.

The Lie?

The point here is to point out just how badly
you have been lied to and hopefully point
you in the correct direction. Thus, despite
the common suggestion, you need not buy
into the suggestion that you must die at one
hundred or even two hundred is not based on
established facts. We are today brain washed
into early death and as a result, our social
institutions and monetary system is aligned
to this and they rely on it happening.

114

In virtually every scientific video here, there
is proven evidence that today's science is in
some way untrue and must in some way
change to comply with the newly
established science and overwhelming
written historical evidence that is unfolding,
some of it has even been documented to
have been hidden away so as to not upset
the established applecart, which must be
turned on its side as we move forward,

So what happens when the people who read
my books begin living

Oldest Civilization?

This is just another example of how far our
history and science is from the truth. Herein
we hear of the Innerton Field which
compromises many of our current held
theories. These discoveries are now dated at
22,000 BC (so far here and possibly
42,000BC). Much of this report does not
hold water in time. I get 80,000BC. If so, it
is far older than currently held. Check it out
with dowsing. The assumption here is that
people were far more ignorant and religious
is wrong compared to where these people
were actually working.
https://www.youtube.com/watch?v=
ImPSfcnlCiY

Here we have walking people of 4million years ago.

https://www.youtube.com/watch?v=U7iu9EU45Yc

I get that they were speaking and were intelligent even though their structure was different than today. The story here is that the transformation was occurring with the Annunachi. This points out what we gave up to become modern man and its the lie that we are told There no human bone in this fossil record. It proves that Darwin was wrong and there was an Annunaki intervention.

Dinosaur Facts

https://www.youtube.com/watch?v=WdqYPjA9VxA

Soft tissue from dinosaur? So people actually could have ridden on dinosaurs. Dinosaur DNA has now been sequenced. Carbon dating is proven wrong if these discoveries and reports are correct. So could dinosaurs have lived millions of years ago? Certainly, one fact does not change the other. https://www.youtube.com/watch?v=SVSx2wTZ3UU

Science hates to ever be disputed with their
current assumptions, So can we live 800 or
even several thousand years and the reports
will remain wrapped up for another hundred
years as the same ridiculous asssump0tions
are held as fact, correct? This is a religion,
not a science or history that masquerades as
truth. How hard is it t rewrite and teach
what we know as current truth?

 This is a nearly totally new, well polished video that is well edited and presented, yet this is only about agreement, not fact. Note that all of these so-called facts are derived from very limited fossils and never do the find any thing other than few limited fossils and none are ever complete. I fact most of these "facts" are derived from a few sketchy details. How is this science? What we know is that there have been many reports by sailors who claim to have encountered them and, of course, we have the Lock Ness Monster which many have reportedly actually seen.. Also, there have been many reports of not only dinosaurs, but also Abominable Snow Men, Big Foot, etc. who many will swear they have encountered first-hand and even repeatedly, yet science cannot prove, so go unnoticed and these encounters even the subject of humor and humiliation. The idea was always to suppress any such discussions and only honor things that are written in stone. So now we have the Annunachi, who are in fact actually described and reported in thousands of documented stone tablets. Given that we accept dinosaurs so readily and even describe there lives and appearances in great detail. Further, it is beyond argument to begin to discredit thousands of stone tablets, my question here is why does the general population know so much about dinosaurs

118

and so little about the Annunachi? *(4:53)* https://www.youtube.com/watch?v=0A-WD-kz-o4 The further key point here is that fossils are very, very rare and yet this is all that we have to base our past historic proofs. Yes, the fossils are solid and beyond argument, but a few speculate based on these rare finds and this is called science. Yes, dinosaurs could actually exist today yet most have died out due to any number of reasons. There is no era in history when live dragons have not been visually reported even though the name dinosaur was only coined in 1842. Finally, with humans, we have no real record and we cannot prove anything from the fossil record when it comes to modern man. If there is no real record, our assumptions as to when we arrived much more wild in speculation than what science tells us. My point from all of this here is that Neanderthals may be here today and never have died out as science presumes. In fact, a fair percentage of people reading this book may well Neanderthal or an Annunaki/ Neanderthal cross and both we know existed or do exist. How would you know? Nothing else explains the many of the key points raised here other than what the clay tablets document. The Mesopotamians did not know who the Annunachi cross bred with really since there was never a distinction

119

between Cro Magnon and Neanderthal in their time.

Ormes and Monatomic Gold (MG)

Today, we can make and buy monatomic gold online and even make it ourselves, but this has been documented in ancient Annunachi texts and much later in OT the bible, so again it is written in stone (fired clay) and proven.

This white MG powder is sound/ gold captured as light also termed as Manna in the bible. This MG is no longer a supposition and not just known in biblical times which are relatively recent where this report begins. In fact, it does not even begin with Sumaria/ Mesopotamia. The important thing here is the message that we are just beginning to recapture the lost knowledge that the Annunachi brought here over some 400,000 years ago. The significant key part of the disclosure that is the MG is a part of our anti-de-aging system presented here. The discussion on the video below regarding de-aging is with regard to telomere length, still not totally documented by science, but almost totally likely at least a measure of aging and possibly a piece of the de-aging puzzle.

Ormes can be based on many minerals and each has anti-aging/ de-aging properties. All are valuable and significant including silver, gold, platinum, and other noble metals, but keep in mind that in ormes is captured vibration that does the work and despite what is reported, you as a spiritual being can capture sound and light. Therefore, we carry antigravity spiritually.

 Below is a very general overview on this topic with many historic references: https://www.youtube.com/watch?v=9jw8CI6eyl0

The reference below are more technical an less broad from an author who makes MG: http://search.hemailaccessonline.com/?uid=72cd844a-6357-43ec-8634-4c0f2a2ed475&uc=20171023&ap=appfocus1&source=googlesearch-googlesearch-v3&page=newtab&implementation_id=email_4.0.17

David Hudson, the guy who discovered Ormes and his discovery: https://www.youtube.com/watch?v=klbJhwxxqDE

The Pineal Gland

People are told that they are spiritual idiots... that they simply die and that is it. This is today's science, the Newtonian "facts" that we are bombarded with today as this Quantum Level is minimized to any degree possible. The Pineal Gland has been seen as the 3rd eye and the center of awareness since man first came here and by the Annunachi prior to that.

Toxins such as Chlorine, Fluorine, Mercury, Sugar and the various others discussed in "It's the Liver Stupid" close off the pineal and decrease your sensitivity to light which as discussed previously begins with Sound which is always there if you focus your attention on it. It is all vibratory beats and your pineal works off of them.

https://video.search.yahoo.com/yhs/search;_ylt=AwrC5pZ_oGZaNxsAk100n

The Wrap

This link as discussed above tell is how all of the key points in this book are pulled together in this final video which basically wraps up many of the points here. Note that no one here concludes any of my key points here, however. This is just one part of my overall premise here, but it is still very important and note that the crystals that run our cars are a part of your own body and you are, thus, a Quantum Being, as I point out herein, with unlimited potential.

Bibliography

Videography/ Bibliography:
My videos that document, explain, prove, and complement this book (search: You Tube/ James Robert Clark Quantum Science or cut and paste the following URLs):
CP4U a QM device as used in a car (our first application):
https://www.youtube.com/watch?v=YFakNUEQoNM
https://www.youtube.com/watch?v=LcWN_DSmIAI
Life Extension Results
https://www.youtube.com/watch?v=DAQ_sdcgaBM
Potential Lifespan
https://www.youtube.com/watch?v=eH_wcdu2u-4
https://www.youtube.com/watch?v=06kXgs00Cxw

An Introduction to Spontaneous Evolution" Bruce H. Lipton, PhD

"Back Hole" Nassim Haramein

"Beyond Pyramid Power," Dr. Patrick Flanagan, PhD
ISBN 0-87516-208-8

"The Biology of Belief" Bruce H. Lipton, PhD
https://www.brucelipton.com/books/biology-of-belief

"White Paper" Dan Nelson, PhD
Https://www.waybackwater.com/dans-white-paper

Books below by James Robert Clark addressing health available in Amazon books:

"It's The Liver Stupid," 5th edition
◆   Paperback: 324 pages
v   Platform; 5th edition (11/19/17)
◆   ISBN-13: 978-1547010493
"Methylation, Awareness and You"
◆   Print Length: 114 pages
◆   Platform; 2nd edition
◆   Publication Date: December 19,
2014
◆   BASIN: B00R8P7R3
"Pretty Fine Sex is Spiritual"
Paperback 182 pages
Platform 1st Edition
ASBN-13 978 1495396741